Magnificent Magnesium

Magnificent Magnesium

Your Essential Key to a Healthy Heart and More

Dennis Goodman, MD, FACC

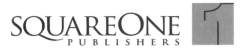

SQUAREONE
PUBLISHERS

The information and advice contained in this book are based upon the research and the personal and professional experiences of the author. They are not intended as a substitute for professional healthcare advice. The publisher and author are not responsible for any adverse effects or consequences resulting from the use of any of the suggestions, preparations, or procedures discussed in this book. All matters pertaining to your physical health should be supervised by a healthcare professional. It is a sign of wisdom, not cowardice, to seek a second or third opinion.

COVER DESIGNER: Jeannie Tudor
TYPESETTER: Gary A. Rosenberg

Square One Publishers
115 Herricks Road
Garden City Park, NY 11040
(516) 535-2010 • (877) 900-BOOK
www.squareonepublishers.com

Library of Congress Cataloging-in-Publication Data
Goodman, Dennis (Dennis A.), author.
  Magnificent magnesium : your essential key to a healthy heart and more / Dennis Goodman, MD.
    pages cm
  Includes bibliographical references and index.
  ISBN 978-0-7570-0391-2
  1. Magnesium in the body. II. Title.
  QP535.M4G6 20214
  612.3'924—dc.
                                  2013030576

Printed in the United States of America

10   9   8   7   6   5   4

Contents

To my parents,
Joe and Muriel Goodman,
and my children,
Adam, Jonathan, and Rebecca,
and to Wendy Fisher.

Acknowledgments

I am deeply appreciative of those who have nurtured, guided, mentored, and supported me throughout my life. Without these wonderful people, this book would not be possible.

I would like to thank my parents, Joe and Muriel Goodman, for inspiring me to always be kind and caring, to be my best self, and for ensuring that I received the very finest education in South Africa—which culminated in the conferment of my medical degree from one of the best universities in the world, the University of Cape Town, South Africa.

Many thanks go to my teachers and mentors in high school and medical school. There is a long list of people to whom I am grateful, but I especially want to acknowledge Norman Sandler, Elliot Wolf, Eddie Tannenbaum, Doc Thomas, and Professors Stuart Saunders, Lionel Opie, Leo Schamroth, Cecil Craig, and Jannie Louw. I was privileged to do my internship at Groote Schuur Hospital in Cape Town, where the first heart transplant was performed by Christian Barnard in 1967. During those years at medical school and internship, away from my hometown of Johannesburg, four wonderful families took me in as one of their own; for this, I thank Dr. Louis and Joan Abramowitz, Harry and Myra Mark, Harry and Pauline Stein, Dov and Bernice Borok, and all their children.

I would like to thank Dr. Philip Troen and Dr. Sheldon Adler of Montefiore Hospital in Pittsburgh, for giving me the opportunity to do my internal medicine residency in the United States and subsequently become a citizen of this great country.

Thanks also to Dr. Robert Roberts, chief of the cardiology department at Baylor College of Medicine, which is associated with Dr. Michael Debakey's cardiac surgery program in Houston, Texas. At Baylor, I received the very best cardiology training. Special thanks to my mentors, Drs. Al Raizner, John Lewis, Jim Young, Craig Pratt, Mario Verani, Phil Henry, Miguel Quinones, William Zoghbi, and the Chapman group.

I would like to thank all my colleagues and friends at Scripps Memorial Hospital and Scripps Clinic—Drs. John Backman, Isaac Bakst, Neil and Ruth Berkowitz, Joel Bernstein, Mark Boiskin, Barry Broomberg, Maurice Buchbinder, Stephen Capon, Martin Charlat, David Dockweiler, Dan Einhorn, Shaun Evans, Ray and Rhona Fink, Carl Fricks, Martin Griglak, Fred Hanson, Wayne Hooper, Paul Hyde, Len Jurkowski, Elizabeth Kaback, Norman Kane, Jurgen Lenz, John Lischke, Mike Mahdavi, Scott McCaul, Lou Katzman, Marc Kramer, Barnie Meltzer, Chris Mende, Frank Meyer, Howard Miller, Ernie Pund, Simon Ritchken, Don Ritt, David Roseman, Mark Sedwitz, Lorna Swartz, Paul Tierstein, Doug Triffon, Sabina Wallach, Pat Wolcott, and the great cardiac surgeons Scott Brewster, Don Buehler, Sasha Giritsky, Richard Stahl, Demetrio Vasquez, and so many others. I particularly want to thank Dr. John Carson, an exceptional human being who exemplifies the values, virtues, and teachings of Sir William Osler.

A special thanks to Gary Fybel, the administrator of Scripps Memorial, and to Susan Taylor, for their enduring friendship and support. Thank you to Irma Flores and Suzi Bustamante for all their help during my tenure as Chief of Cardiology at Scripps Memorial. And many thanks to my incredible office manager, Debbie Heggins, and nurse practitioner, Robin Whitman, who worked with me for over twenty years.

Thanks to Mimi Guarnieri and Rauni King, who put me on the path to becoming a truly integrative physician. I learned so much from them and their great team at the Scripps Center for Integrative Medicine.

My thanks also go to Drs. Glenn Fishman and Norma Keller, who gave me the opportunity to work and teach as a cardiologist at one of the great medical institutions of the world, New York University Langone Medical Center. Thanks to the great staff and my wonderful partners at New York Medical Associates, Drs. Mark Lipton, Stanley Schrem, and Jeffrey Kohn. I am indebted to Drs. Frank Lipman, Daryl Isaacs, Florence Comite, Keith Berkowitz, Leah Lagos, and Marnie Potash for their unwavering support.

I am grateful to Larry Trivieri and Morley Robbins (the "Magnesium Man") for being such fantastic resources and providing me with so much detailed information on magnesium. Their help with this book has been invaluable. Morley's selfless passion and commitment to bringing the multitude of benefits of magnesium to the general public are unparalleled.

Thanks to the staff at Square One Publishers—to my publisher, Rudy Shur, who has been a rock of Gibraltar with his wisdom and support throughout the process, and my editor, Miye Bromberg, for her never-ending willingness to help.

I thank Drs. Norman Kane, Norman Gordon, Mike Forman, and Jim Adams; Gershon Jaffe; Mike, Patti, and Russel Hoffman; Rob Martin; Bob Austen; Dean Draznin; and Terri Slater; they have provided a wealth of knowledge and friendship.

Huge thanks to my special partner, Wendy Fisher, who has encouraged and supported me through all the many hours of researching and writing this book.

Thanks to my mother and my sisters, Myra Salkinder and Elaine Lucey—thanks to all my family. I am so fortunate to have their constant love and support.

Enormous thanks to my incredible children—Adam, my daughter-in-law Anat, Jonathan, and Rebecca—as well as to their wonderful mother, Tanya. Additional thanks to Adam and Jonathan for all their editing and research help along the way.

Lastly, I want to thank all of the patients I have treated over my twenty-five years in practice. They have given me so much pleasure and the greatest gift of all—a meaningful life and the opportunity to make a small difference in the world.

Magnificent Magnesium

Introduction

All too often, the public is besieged by reports that a particular supplement holds the secret to a longer, healthier life. Exciting new information is released, spurring a surge of interest and, of course, a rise in supplement sales. As claims about the nutrient circulate, people are exposed to some truth, some hype, and, often, a good deal of wishful thinking. The pity is that while the media focuses on a short-lived trend, some very important nutrients are often overlooked—to the detriment of everyone's health.

Consider the following: Heart disease is the number one killer in the United States today. Each year, we spend billions of dollars on medical tests, operations, hospital stays, rehab centers, equipment, and drugs—all to help prevent or remedy heart disease—yet with very little to show for our investments. Heart disease accounts for direct and indirect costs of more than $190.3 billion each year, and the American Heart Association forecasts that these costs will increase by a minimum of 200 percent over the next twenty years.

Billions more go to the satellite industries that have developed to cater to our health epidemics, producing everything from best-selling diet books to weight loss centers to lines of "heart-healthy" foods and making promises that they can prevent or reverse these conditions. The media is flooded with ads and television shows that tell us that if we don't do something, we are bound to become statistics—the victims of our own inaction. Yet there *is* something we can do to offset the outrageous expenditures and unnecessary procedures; in fact, there's something we can take even now to help prevent these life-threatening health conditions from developing in the first place. The answer is simple, inexpensive, and effective: magnesium.

As a heart specialist, I feel that the treasures held within magnesium have yet to be embraced by the medical community. The more studies I read confirming the vital roles magnesium plays in the body, the more clearly I realize that too few people know how critical magnesium is to good health.

Magnesium is the eighth most abundant element on Earth and the eleventh most common element in the human body. It has been studied by medical researchers for over a hundred years, and while it has always been considered a reasonably important mineral, it is, in fact, essential to the proper functioning of the body. This master mineral is a necessary ingredient for approximately three hundred and fifty enzyme systems, thus playing a role in the majority of your body's metabolic processes. Surprisingly, however, upwards of 80 percent of Americans are deficient in this nutrient.

Why is magnesium deficiency worth our attention? First and foremost, without the proper levels of magnesium in the body, we are subject to heart attacks—the number one killer of Americans—as well as a variety of other heart-related disorders. Second, many other serious health problems are associated with magnesium deficiency, including type 2 diabetes, metabolic syndrome, osteoporosis, muscle cramps, fatigue, depression, migraines, and insomnia.

At this point, you may be wondering, "If magnesium is this important, why haven't I heard about it before?" While there are many reasons why magnesium has been overlooked for so long, I strongly believe that magnesium's time is now. Once you have read this book, you will understand the difference magnesium can make in your life. The goal of *Magnificent Magnesium* is to contribute to wider public knowledge about the value of this mineral—knowledge that you will be able to apply the moment you turn the book's last page.

This book is designed to present an understanding of magnesium with a sharp focus on its role in heart health and several other aspects of physical well-being. Chapter 1 takes an unflinching look at the heart disease epidemic that claimed nearly 800,000 American lives in 2010, with stroke killing over 129,000 people that same year. It examines the most common forms of heart disease and details their causes, risk factors, symptoms, diagnoses, and typical treatment methods, so that you will be able to recognize and potentially prevent these devastating conditions.

In Chapter 2, you will be introduced to magnesium and its many roles in supporting and maintaining your body's vital functions. You will also learn the reason that magnesium deficiency is so common in the United States today: stress. Stress comes in many forms—psychological, physical, and environmental. The important thing to understand is that all of these forms of stress contribute to the extensive depletion of magnesium from our bodies and food sources.

Chapter 3 sets the foundation for understanding heart disease, providing an overview of the cardiovascular system. By learning how your heart and blood vessels work under normal circumstances, you will be able to understand what happens when something goes wrong—as with the heart conditions discussed in Chapter 1. This knowledge base also allows you to see how magnesium can help your body, from the cellular level on up.

In Chapter 4, you will take a closer look at the way the medical community currently views and treats heart disease. The chapter also introduces an emerging model for understanding heart disease—and preventing it. The starved heart model of heart disease asserts that without an optimal supply of magnesium, the heart begins to break down at every level, leading to energy starvation, dysfunction, and eventually cardiovascular disease. Accordingly, to reverse or protect against cardiovascular disease, it is essential to maintain good magnesium levels and excellent magnesium stores.

Chapter 5 demonstrates that the benefits of magnesium

extend far beyond their applications for cardiovascular disease. Many of the United States' other major health conditions are caused or exacerbated by magnesium deficiency. This chapter lays out the research, showing that you can help improve, protect against, and even prevent these diseases by simply increasing your intake of magnesium.

Finally, in Chapter 6, all this information is put to work, providing you with a practical guide to integrating magnesium into your life. You will be shown how to determine the amount of magnesium you need to obtain and maintain optimal wellness, taking into account your current magnesium status and the amount you burn through on a day-to-day basis. You will also be provided with information on the best sources for getting this vital nutrient, so that you will never be without.

By the time you finish reading *Magnificent Magnesium,* you will be equipped with the knowledge you need to understand the origins of heart disease—and, potentially, to prevent it from ever developing. But while reading this book is a significant first step, it is far more important that you actually use the tools contained within to take charge of your health. Be proactive; only you can change your life!

1

What's Our Problem?

Heart disease is the leading cause of mortality in the United States, accounting for 25 percent of all recorded deaths. It strikes indiscriminately—teenagers and adults, men and women, blacks and whites—all are susceptible. It can kill quickly or it can linger for years, causing pain, depression, and a wide variety of painful and debilitating symptoms. Affecting over 80 million Americans today, heart disease is a modern-day plague with a reach and severity that extend further with every passing week. And yet, for the most part, too many of us simply accept it as the price we pay to live in a country of so-called abundance. But it is a very high price.

So if we know we have a problem, why does heart disease persist? Is it genetics, our diet, or just a lack of exercise? Is it our cholesterol levels or blood pressure? Why is it that there are so many seemingly right answers, and yet, so many of us continue to die prematurely? This book attempts to address all of these issues, and to present an answer of its own. There is a solution to our health woes, a tragically underutilized remedy that has been with us for decades: magnesium.

In order to get a sense of just how fully magnesium can improve our quality of life, we need to examine the epidemic that poses the greatest challenge to our health: heart disease. Moreover, we need to know the ways in which this epidemic has typically been addressed by the medical community. An understanding of the types and causes of heart disease, and the standard medical responses to them, will enable you to make better decisions regarding your own well-being.

THE STATISTICS TELL A TALE

Since the beginning of the twentieth century, heart disease has been our nation's number one killer. It is unlikely to give up that position any time soon. Consider these grim statistics from the American Heart Association's *Heart Disease and Stroke Statistics— 2013 Update:*

- More than 2,150 Americans die of heart disease each and every day. That's an average of one death every 39 seconds.

- An average of 150,000 Americans who die of heart disease each year are younger than 65 years of age, while 33 percent of all deaths caused by heart disease occur before the age of 75 years, which is well below the average life expectancy of 77.9 years.

- Coronary heart disease causes one of every six deaths in the United States each year, while one out of every eighteen deaths is caused by stroke.

- An average of 800,000 Americans die of heart disease each year.

- Each year, an estimated 785,000 Americans have a heart attack, and 470,000 more have a repeat attack.

- Approximately 195,000 Americans experience their first silent (unnoticed or undiagnosed) heart attacks each year.

- Approximately every 25 seconds, an American will have a coronary event, and approximately every minute, someone will die of one.

Once mistakenly thought to primarily affect men, approximately half of all deaths caused by heart disease in the United States each year occur among women, accounting for more than six times the number of deaths caused by breast cancer. Although mortality rates caused by heart disease have started to decline over the past fifty years, the overall toll continues to rise, both in terms of impaired health and financial cost.

Here is the most important statistic to remember: For half of the people who die of a heart attack, death is the first and last symptom that they ever experience. In other words, prior to their deaths, most victims never experienced any sort of symptom to warn them that they were at risk for heart attack. This is why it is so important to work regularly with your physician to determine your risk and monitor the health of your heart and overall cardiovascular system.

THE MOST COMMON TYPES OF HEART DISEASE

We can certainly see the devastation that cardiovascular disease produces. In order to understand the different ways that cardiovascular disease affects us, let's take a closer look at the fifteen most common types. They include:

- Angina Pectoris
- Arrhythmias/Atrial Fibrillation (Irregular Heartbeat)
- Atherosclerosis
- Cardiac Arrest
- Congestive Heart Failure
- Coronary Heart Disease (CHD)
- Enlarged Heart (Cardiomegaly)
- Heart Attack (Acute Myocardial Infarction)
- Heart Murmur
- Heart Muscle Disease (Cardiomyopathy)
- High Blood Pressure (Hypertension)
- Mitral Valve Prolapse

- Pericarditis/Pericardial Effusion

- Premature Ventricular Contraction (PVC)

- Stroke

This section will define what each condition is, explain why it occurs, describe its symptoms, and explain how it is currently diagnosed and treated.

Angina Pectoris

The term angina pectoris is derived from Latin and means "squeezing of the chest." Angina is chest pain caused by a decreased supply of blood to the heart muscle, usually due to a lesion on the walls or valves or the heart, or because of a narrowing of the coronary arteries. As a result of this constriction or blockage, the heart receives less oxygen—a condition called *ischemia.* Spasms of the coronary arteries can also be involved.

Risk factors for angina pectoris include smoking, lack of exercise, chronic stress, and high blood pressure. Being overweight or obese also increases risk, as does diabetes. The risk for angina also increases as you age.

Classical or typical symptoms of angina include pain, pressure, or other discomfort in the middle of the chest. This chest pain can radiate to the throat, jaw, upper back, arms, and even teeth. Unfortunately, cases of angina often go misdiagnosed or undiagnosed in women, who are more likely to suffer atypical symptoms, including palpitations, dizziness, heartburn, indigestion, nausea, numbness in the arms, weakness, and shortness of breath. Symptoms typically worsen after a heavy meal or physical exertion, and during times of emotional stress, as all of these situations demand that more oxygen be pumped to the heart.

There are two types of angina: stable and unstable. Stable angina is the most common type, and is characterized by typical symptoms that are predictable. Ordinarily, symptoms last around five minutes or so, and then subside.

Unstable angina is a more serious condition, with symptoms being more severe and less predictable, and usually lasting much longer. Unstable angina symptoms can occur even at times of rest. Because unstable angina is often a precursor and warning sign of a heart attack, prompt medical attention should be sought at the first sign of unstable angina.

Angina can be diagnosed using a number of tools. An electrocardiogram (EKG), which records the electrical activity of heart, can detect signs of ischemia and is also useful for monitoring changes to the heart muscle caused by a lack of oxygen. Even when EKG readings are normal, however, angina may still be present. Physicians who suspect that this is the case may also use exercise stress testing, in which a patient is asked to perform activities that stress the heart (such as walking on a treadmill or using a stationary bike) while their EKG readings are continuously monitored.

If the exercise stress test remains inconclusive, your physician may order a stress echocardiogram or nuclear heart scan. Stress echocardiography combines ultrasound imaging of the heart muscle with exercise stress testing in order to screen for abnormalities in your heart's contractions. Since there is no radiation exposure, stress echocardiography is preferred to nuclear heart scans. In a nuclear heart scan, a safe, radioactive trace substance such as thallium or Cardiolite is injected into your bloodstream and an external camera is used to monitor the activity of this trace substance as it travels through your veins to your heart. Typically, there are two parts to this test; one set of images will be taken after a mild stress test (similar to the one described above), and another set will be produced later, when your body is at rest. Both these tests allow your physician to see how well blood is flowing through your heart, and can identify any muscle areas that might be damaged or narrowed.

If your stress test yields abnormal results, your doctor may also order a coronary computed tomography angiogram (CTA). This test uses a computed tomography (CT) scan to visually track the progress of an intravenous dye containing iodine through the bloodstream, making it possible to see the coronary arteries and determine if any blockages are present. For most patients, a CTA is an excellent, noninvasive way to diagnose angina.

In some cases, cardiologists may also order or perform a cardiac catheterization with angiography. During this procedure, small, hollow plastic tubes (catheters) are inserted through arteries in the groin or forearm and threaded into the openings of the coronary arteries under the guidance of X-rays. Iodine contrast dye is injected into the arteries while an X-ray video is recorded, providing doctors with images of the location and severity of coronary artery disease. Cardiac catheterization is commonly regarded as the most accurate test to detect coronary artery narrowing. It is particularly useful in cases where there is a high likelihood that therapeutic intervention will be required, because it allows for immediate treatment. If a blocked artery is found, a metal tube called a stent can be placed inside the troubled area, supporting the artery and facilitating blood flow.

If angina symptoms are present but not severe, or if no serious blockages are seen on a CTA or cardiac catheterization, doctors may simply instruct their patients to make healthy lifestyle changes. With better food choices, smaller meals, rest, and stress reduction, many patients will see their symptoms improve. Otherwise, medical treatments may be advised. Treatment options include conventional medications, such as nitroglycerin tablets or sprays to reduce the heart muscle's demand for oxygen; beta blockers, to reduce the effects of adrenaline on the heart; and calcium channel blockers, to lower blood pressure and reduce the pumping force of the heart muscle, and thus its need for oxygen.

If the above measures fail to correct the problem, angina patients may be advised to consider surgery. In addition to the stent placement described above, the two most common surgical procedures for angina pectoris are angioplasty and coronary artery bypass surgery. During an angioplasty, a small balloon is inserted into the narrowed artery and inflated; this dilates the narrowed artery and allows blood to flow more freely. In some cases, a small mesh tube, or stent, may also be placed inside the artery to hold it open. Coronary artery bypass surgery, a form of open heart surgery, is a procedure that redirects blood around a blocked artery (bypassing it), creating a new pathway for blood to flow to and from the heart. This is done by taking an artery or vein from the patient's leg or chest wall and sewing one end above the blocked coronary artery and the other end below the blockage.

Regardless of the type of surgery performed, angina patients are still vulnerable to future heart attack. It is therefore essential that all angina sufferers make the necessary lifestyle changes to lower their risk, following a heart-friendly diet, maintaining a healthy weight, exercising regularly, reducing stress, and keeping appropriate levels of cholesterol and blood sugar.

Arrhythmia/Atrial Fibrillation

Arrhythmia is a condition characterized by an abnormal or irregular heartbeat caused by faulty electrical impulses to the heart. Unlike other organs and muscles in your body, your heart has its own "electrical generator"—a specialized group of cells located in the heart's upper right chamber (right atrium). As you'll read in Chapter 3, this group of cells, known as the sinoatrial (SA) node, creates a series of electrical impulses that make your heart pump blood in an even, continuous flow. Arrhythmia occurs either when the SA node is damaged or when there is some other disruption to the heart's conduction of electrical signals (see page 78 for more information). There are two basic kinds of irregular heart rhythms. The first is known as *bradycardia,* and is characterized by heartbeats that are too slow—fewer than sixty beats per minute. The second type is known as *tachycardia,* and is characterized by a racing heartbeat of more than 100 beats per minute.

The most common form of arrhythmia is *atrial fibrillation* (AF), in which the heart's two top chambers (the atria) beat quickly and irregularly, causing blood to pool within and preventing the atria from working in harmony with the heart's lower two chambers (the ventricles). According to the Centers for Disease Control and Prevention (CDC), approximately 2.66 million people currently suffer from atrial fibrillation, and as many as 12 million people will have the condition by 2050. Less common, but very serious, are the two forms of arrhythmia that occur in the lower two chambers (ventricles) of the heart: *ventricular tachycardia* and *ventricular fibrillation*. The result of these two conditions is that the ventricles are unable to pump blood to the rest of your body. Your blood pressure drops, and your vital organs cease to receive the blood they need to operate. Ventricular arrhythmias are the most common cause of death related to heart attack. Immediate attention— cardiopulmonary resuscitation (CPR) and/or defibrillation—is necessary to prevent death.

A number of factors can increase the risk of arrhythmia, including high blood pressure, smoking, excessive alcohol consumption, and the use of pharmaceutical drugs, including over-the-counter cold and flu medications. Other risk factors include sleep apnea (a condition in which breathing is interrupted during sleep), thyroid problems, and other pre-existing heart conditions (including coronary artery disease, heart valve problems, and congestive heart failure).

Symptoms of arrhythmia can often go undetected, manifesting as a brief and barely noticeable skipped heartbeat. In more serious cases, where arrhythmia prevents the heart from pumping enough blood, patients can feel sensations of fluttering in the chest or neck, along with dizziness or lightheadedness, fatigue, and fainting. Other symptoms include chest pain and shortness of breath. If you experience any of these symptoms, contact your physician or seek medical help immediately. In some cases, arrhythmia can trigger a heart attack and even cause death.

Arrhythmia is most often detected with an electrocardiogram (EKG), which also helps physicians determine where in the heart the problem starts. Stress testing and tilt table tests (used to detect the cause of arrhythmia-induced fainting) are also commonly used, as are tests that specifically map the heart's electrical system and any flaws that may have arisen in it, including electrophysiology studies (EP studies). During an EP study, thin, flexible catheters with electrodes on their tips are threaded through the heart's blood vessels in order to provide a precise picture of the pathways that electrical impulses take while traveling through the heart. The electrodes can also be used either to trigger or to stabilize an arrhythmia, enabling the doctor to pinpoint the exact location of the problem.

If an arrhythmia is detected, your doctor may ask you to alter your lifestyle with an improved diet, exercise, and stress management. Medications may also be prescribed in order to control arrhythmia directly, or to deal with associated risks; anticoagulants (blood thinners, beta blockers, and calcium channel and/or sodium channel blockers) are all commonly used. Should all of these options fail, other treatment options may be required.

The most common nondrug procedures used to treat arrhythmia are cardioversion, defibrillation, cardiac ablation, and the Maze procedure. Cardioversion is used to temporarily normalize arrhythmias that could otherwise cause heart attack or death. Using either fast-acting drugs or an electric shock delivered with defibrillator paddles directly over the heart, the abnormal heartbeat is interrupted, allowing the heart's electrical system to regain control and restore a normal heart rhythm. Defibrillation is a somewhat more intense form of cardioversion that is performed in emergency situations involving severe or highly irregular arrhythmias, as in cardiac arrest; it employs a stronger set of electrical shocks to jolt the heart rhythm back to normal.

In some cases of tachycardia and ventricular fibrillation, an electrical device known as an implantable cardioverter defibrillator (ICD) may be surgically inserted into a patient's chest, as a pacemaker might be. When an arrythmia occurs, the ICD delivers a shock to reset the heartbeat and get the SA node to send a normal electrical signal. (See the inset on page 79 for more information.)

In severe cases of arrhythmia, physicians may elect to perform more invasive surgical procedures to remove damaged or otherwise abnormal tissue in the heart muscle that is triggering arrhythmia. During cardiac ablation, a thin tube (catheter) is inserted into a vein and then guided into the heart muscle. Once there, the tip of the catheter emits a burst of energy to destroy the areas of heart tissue shown to be causing abnormal electrical signals.

The Maze procedure is an invasive surgical procedure used to treat atrial fibrillation. During the Maze procedure, the surgeon makes a number of incisions, which are then sewn up again, creating scar tissue. These scars serve as barriers, forcing the electrical impulses responsible for your heartbeat to travel along a single, uniform pathway into the ventricles so that a normal heart rhythm can be restored.

Atherosclerosis

Atherosclerosis refers to a hardening or blockage of the arteries due to the accumulation of a waxy substance called plaque. Plaque builds up as part of your body's inflammatory response to damage in the walls of the arteries. When your arteries are damaged as the result of high blood pressure, cigarette smoke, environmental toxins, or the presence of other irritants, your body sends cholesterol and other substances to the wound in an attempt to repair it. Collectively, these fatty deposits are known as plaque. Over time, they can build up, narrowing and hardening the arteries, and thus reducing the flow of blood and increasing blood pressure levels. (For a more complete explanation of how atherosclerosis develops, see Chapter 4.)

Risk factors for atherosclerosis include age, diabetes and insulin resistance, high blood pressure, high cholesterol, obesity, smoking, and a family history of heart disease. Because inflammation is an integral part of the process by which atherosclerosis develops, doctors have theorized that factors that increase inflammation can often indirectly contribute to atherosclerosis, too. For example, several studies have shown that there was a strong association between atherosclerosis and *Chlamydophila pneumoniae,* one of the bacteria that causes pneumonia. Scientists theorized that because *C. pneumoniae* infections seemed to cause or contribute to the inflammation that in turn causes atherosclerosis, treating the infections with antibiotics would potentially help reduce the atherosclerosis. Unfortunately, subsequent studies showed that patients with atherosclerosis derived no overall benefit from antibiotics, and the theory was deemed less plausible.

Atherosclerosis can go undetected for years before symptoms present themselves. In fact, in recent years, an alarming number of teens and preteens have been found to have some degree of atherosclerotic plaques. Overall, nearly 5 million Americans are diagnosed with atherosclerosis each year, while a significantly higher number of Americans have already been diagnosed and are living with this condition.

Symptoms of atherosclerosis depend on the extent of the blockage and the specific arteries affected. In arteries of the heart, atherosclerosis can manifest as chest pain or pressure (angina), while in leg or arm arteries atherosclerosis can cause intermittent pain. In the arteries that lead into the brain, atherosclerosis can produce warning signs of stroke, including slurred speech, drooping muscles in the face, and numbness or weakness in the arms or legs. In arteries leading to the genitals, atherosclerosis can cause erectile dysfunction in men, while in women, the same condition can reduce blood flow to the vagina, resulting in less pleasurable sex. Unfortunately, many patients will not show symptoms until the atherosclerosis is severe, blocking over 70 percent of the affected artery. This makes atherosclerosis harder to diagnose and treat.

Blood tests that screen for LDL ("bad") cholesterol, HDL ("good") cholesterol, and total cholesterol levels—as well as other markers such as homocysteine, C-reactive protein (CRP), and lipoprotein-associated phospholipase (Lp-PLA-2)—can indicate whether atherosclerosis is likely to be present. Other diagnostic tests include the various forms of stress testing, although these methods have certain drawbacks. Stress tests only detect large blockages that have obstructed at least 70 percent of your arterial passage. Accordingly, you can still be at serious risk for heart attack even if your doctor says you "passed a stress test." Your arteries may not be severely blocked, but they may not necessarily be clean and healthy, either.

Fortunately, there are more effective and noninvasive tests that can detect plaque in the coronary or carotid (neck) arteries before a significant blockage develops. Two of the most common procedures used for early detection of atherosclerosis—that is, before most symptoms arise—are coronary calcium scoring by CT scan, which measures the amount of plaque in your coronary arteries, and carotid intima-media thickness testing (CIMT), which uses ultrasound technology to screen your carotid arteries for plaque.

Should atherosclerosis be detected, your doctor may prescribe aspirin or cholesterol-lowering drugs—statins or other natural alternatives. You will probably be asked to make certain lifestyle changes, involving a low-cholesterol diet, regular exercise, and the avoidance of unhealthy behaviors such as smoking and alcohol consumption. Because stress is a major risk factor for heart disease, learning to reduce or control it is essential for the proper treatment of atherosclerosis, as you will read later in this chapter. By adopting these lifestyle changes, you can prevent plaque from developing or progressing, significantly reducing the likelihood that atherosclerosis will threaten your life.

Cardiac Arrest

Cardiac arrest, also known as cardiopulmonary or circulatory arrest, sudden cardiac arrest, and sudden cardiac death, is a condition in which the heart abruptly stops beating. Cardiac arrest differs from heart attack in that the disruption of blood flow is caused not by a physical blockage, but rather by an electrical disturbance that impairs the heart's ability to pump blood to the rest of the body. And while the heart may continue to beat during a heart attack, it stops completely in cardiac arrest. As a result, blood ceases to flow, preventing oxygen from being delivered to the body and brain. Cardiac arrest is a very serious medical emergency. Each year, an estimated 295,000 Americans suffer cardiac arrest; only 8 percent will survive when the incident occurs out of hospital. The majority of cases that are not treated within ten minutes end in death; patients who survive are likely to suffer brain damage due to the loss of blood flow and needed oxygen to the brain.

The immediate cause of cardiac arrest is usually a severe arrhythmia such as ventricular fibrillation (see page 11), in which the heartbeat cycle is electrically disrupted to the point of stopping altogether. But this life-threatening arrhythmia is itself the result of an underlying heart condition, usually coronary artery disease, although occasionally an enlarged and weakened heart (cardiomyopathy), heart valve disease, or congenital heart defect is to blame. Cardiac arrest can also be caused by noncardiovascular sources, including trauma, gastrointestinal bleeding, or hemorrhaging inside the cranium. Other factors that compound the increase the risk of cardiac arrest include age (the risk increases in men over forty-five and women over fifty-five), smoking, high blood pressure, being overweight or obese, lack of exercise, diabetes, excessive alcohol consumption, drug use, and a previous history of heart disease. Men are two to three times more at risk for cardiac arrest than women, and blacks are about one-third as likely as other groups to survive.

Symptoms of cardiac arrest appear suddenly and must be treated immediately. A victim of cardiac arrest will collapse, unconscious, unable to breathe, and with no pulse. Sometimes cardiac arrest will be preceded by a period of faintness or dizziness, chest pains, shortness of breath, nausea, or vomiting. It is essential that these symptoms be taken seriously.

Due to the catastrophic nature of cardiac arrest, immediate treatment is essential for survival. A patient is more likely to die with every moment that passes without medical treatment. If you or someone near you appears to be suffering a cardiac arrest, call 911 immediately. Until emergency medical treatment is available, perform cardiopulmonary resuscitation (CPR). If you have not been trained in basic CPR, now is the time to learn—you never know when you could be called on to save a life. Contact your local American Heart Association office for more information. Even if you don't know CPR, you can still assist the patient until help arrives by pushing firmly and steadily on the patient's chest at a rate of around 100 pushes per minute. Allow the chest to fully rise between each push. Continue until help arrives or until the patient regains consciousness and is able to breathe unaided.

As soon as possible, an automated external defibrillator (AED) should be used to deliver electrical shocks to the patient's heart in an effort to get it beating normally again. Many public spaces—including shopping malls, hotels, convention centers, airports, and sports stadiums—have AEDs for general use. If one is not immediately available, the police or emergency medical staff will provide one when they arrive at the scene. When the patient gets to the emergency room, drugs will be administered in order to treat a heart attack (if one has occurred), stabilize heart rhythm, and rectify an electrolyte imbalance.

The cause of cardiac arrest is diagnosed after the event. Patients who survive cardiac arrest need to be tested in order to identify the underlying factors that triggered the episode, which, if left unaddressed, could trigger future episodes. Testing methods include electrocardiogram (EKG), echocardiogram, chest X-ray, and angiogram. Blood and hormone testing are also commonly ordered. Other tests include computed tomography (CT) scan, magnetic resonance imaging (MRI), ejection fraction testing, nuclear heart scans, and electrophysiology (EP) studies.

Treatment may include medications, including angiotensin-converting enzyme (ACE) inhibitors, which widen and relax the blood vessels; beta blockers; and calcium channel blockers. Surgery may also be recommended in order to prevent future recurrence of cardiac arrest. Surgical methods can range from the implantation of an implantable cardioverter defibrillator (ICD) device to monitor heart rhythm and reset it, if necessary; coronary angioplasty stenting or bypass surgery; or corrective heart surgery to repair faulty heart valves, diseased heart muscle tissue, or congenital heart deformities. A procedure called radiofrequency catheter ablation can also be used in order to destroy (ablate) the area or areas of the heart that are causing the arrhythmia.

Because cardiac arrest is frequently fatal, prevention is often the best cure. If you are at risk, your doctor may advise you to make lifestyle changes in order to lower your chance of cardiac arrest. Don't smoke, drink moderately or not at all, eat a balanced diet, and get plenty of exercise; these choices will improve your health and help lower your vulnerability to cardiac arrest.

Congestive Heart Failure

Congestive heart failure (CHF) is a condition in which the heart is unable to pump a sufficient supply of blood to the rest of the body. CHF can be either chronic and ongoing or sudden and acute. Most cases of CHF initially develop in the heart's main blood pumping chamber, the left ventricle. CHF gets its name because when it occurs, blood backs up into, or congests, the liver, abdomen, lungs, and/or legs, ankles, and feet. Left untreated, CHF can cause heart valve problems, heart attack, stroke, and damage to the liver and kidneys.

CHF can be caused by a variety of conditions that weaken or damage the heart, including coronary heart disease, heart attack, high blood pressure, congenital heart defects (heart abnormalities that are present from birth), damaged heart muscle or valves, inflammation of the heart, arrhythmia, and atherosclerosis. Risk for CHF can be increased by various noncardiovascular diseases, including severe anemia, diabetes and certain diabetes medications, hyperthyroidism and hypothyroidism, emphysema, lupus, infections, kidney disease, blood clots in the lungs, smoking, and excessive alcohol consumption.

There are many symptoms of CHF, ranging from chest pain and shortness of breath (after exertion or when lying down), fatigue, weakness, edema (swelling in ankles, feet, or legs), rapid or irregular heartbeat, swelling in the abdomen, sudden weight gain due to fluid retention, and nausea. All of these symptoms are typically more severe in cases of sudden CHF.

Diagnosis of CHF begins with a thorough medical history intake and physical exam. Often, your doctor will order a blood test to screen for a chemical known as brain natriuretic peptide, or BNP, high levels of which can indicate CHF. Other diagnostic methods include chest X-ray, electrocardiogram (EKG), echocardiogram, computed tomography (CT) scan, magnetic resonance imaging (MRI), and stress testing. An ejection fraction test can also be used, usually in conjunction with an echocardiogram. An ejection fraction measures how well your heart pumps blood. In a healthy heart, the ejection fraction is above 55 percent, meaning that more than half of all the blood that fills the ventricle is pumped out with each heartbeat; a reading lower than 50 percent can confirm heart failure. Lung function will likely also be checked through the use of a stethoscope to listen for signs of lung congestion.

Chronic CHF requires lifelong management. With proper treatment, CHF symptoms can improve; in some cases the heart itself can even become stronger over time. Conventional medications used to treat CHF include angiotensin-converting enzyme (ACE) inhibitors and angiotensin receptor blockers, both of which widen blood vessels, reduce blood pressure, and improve blood flow; digoxin (digitalis), which increases heart muscle contractions and slows the heartbeat; beta blockers, which slow heart rate and reduce blood pressure; and diuretics, to decrease fluid buildup.

Surgical procedures to treat CHF include coronary bypass surgery, heart valve repair or replacement, placement of an implantable cardioverter defibrillator, the implantation of a mechanical heart pump, and the insertion of a pacemaker. In severe cases of CHF, a heart transplant may be warranted.

Patients with CHF are often advised to weigh themselves each morning and to notify their doctors if they experience a weight gain of three pounds or more over a 24-hour period. Such weight gain is usually a sign of fluid retention, indicating the need for adjusted treatment. CHF patients are also advised to achieve and maintain a healthy weight; follow a low-fat, low-salt diet; and limit their intake of alcohol and, in more severe cases, other fluids.

Coronary Heart Disease

Coronary heart disease (CHD), also called coronary artery disease, is a type of atherosclerosis that occurs specifically in the arteries of the heart. Once the inner wall of a coronary artery becomes diseased or damaged, fatty deposits composed of cholesterol and other cellular waste products—plaque—accumulate in the coronary artery walls, hardening and narrowing these vessels and restricting blood flow. Because the coronary arteries are already narrower than your other arteries, the effects of this particular type of atherosclerosis can be serious: Deprived of blood, your heart can simply stop working. According to the CDC, an estimated 6 percent of all American adults suffer from CHD, many of them unknowingly.

As with atherosclerosis, CHD can be caused by a variety of factors, including poor diet and lack of exercise, high blood pressure, smoking, chronic stress, high levels of LDL ("bad") cholesterol and low levels of HDL ("good") cholesterol, and other health conditions, including diabetes, sleep apnea, and obesity. Radiation therapy, especially when used to treat certain cancers, can also cause CHD.

Initially, symptoms of CHD may not be apparent, but as the condition worsens, so, too, do the symptoms. As the artery blockages grow, CHD can manifest as angina (chest pain), and shortness of breath. Left untreated, CHD can result in arrhythmia, heart muscle failure, heart attack, or sudden death.

Because CHD is a "silent" killer—meaning you can suffer from the disease without experiencing any of its symptoms—regular medical checkups are important for everyone, but especially for those who are considered to have a higher risk for developing this serious disease. A physical exam and a blood test will provide general screening for CHD. Your doctor may also order additional diagnostic tests, such as an electrocardiogram (EKG), echocardiogram, and a stress test. In cases of CHD where significant blockages are suspected, other tests may be prescribed, such as a computed tomography (CT) scan, angiogram, or magnetic resonance angiogram (MRA), during which magnetic resonance imaging (MRI) is used to track the progress of an injected contrast dye in order to check for areas of the arteries that may be narrowed or blocked.

Treatment for CHD usually involves a combination of drugs and lifestyle changes, including adopting a heart-healthy diet, regular exercise, stress management, the cessation of smoking, and often weight loss. The most commonly used drugs to treat CHD are aspirin, statins, beta blockers, calcium channel blockers, and ACE inhibitors. In some cases, nitroglycerin tablets, patches, or sprays may also be used to control chest pain related to CHD, and to help widen arteries. If a nonpharmacological approach is warranted, the most common procedures are angioplasty and coronary bypass surgery (see pages 10 and 11).

Enlarged Heart

Enlarged heart, or cardiomegaly, is not a disease, but rather a manifestation of another heart condition, such as coronary artery disease, high blood pressure, heart valve disease, arrhythmia, or a weakened or damaged heart muscle. While an enlarged heart is usually a chronic condition, there are also more temporary situations in which the heart becomes enlarged for a short period of time due to pregnancy, excessive exertion, or stress being placed on the body. The risk of developing an enlarged heart increases for anyone born with a condition that affects the structure of the heart (congenital heart disease), and for people with high blood pressure or a family history of enlarged heart.

An enlarged heart can go unnoticed, with no signs that anything is wrong; alternatively, it can present with symptoms such as arrhythmia, chest pain, coughing, edema, difficulty exercising, and shortness of breath. Left untreated, an enlarged heart can result in blood clots within the heart chambers, heart failure, cardiac arrest, and sudden death.

Physicians use a variety of diagnostic methods to screen for an enlarged heart. These include electrocardiogram (EKG), echocardiogram, chest X-ray, computed tomography (CT) scan, magnetic resonance imaging (MRI), and stress testing. In addition, blood tests will usually be ordered to screen for signs of other possible heart problems.

If detected early, an enlarged heart can be treated and even reversed. Treatment options include medications such as angiotensin-converting enzyme (ACE) inhibitors, anticoagulants (blood thinners), beta blockers, diuretics, and digoxin (digitalis). Surgery may also be necessary. Surgical options include the placement of an implantable cardioverter device (ICD) or ventricular assist device (VAD), heart valve surgery, and coronary bypass.

Heart Attack (Acute Myocardial Infarction)

A heart attack, or acute myocardial infarction (AMI), occurs when blood flow to the heart is interrupted, causing heart muscle cells to die. Lack of blood flow to the heart is most often due to a blockage of a coronary artery caused by a substance called *vulnerable plaque*. Vulnerable plaque is an unstable combination of cholesterol, fatty acids, and white blood cells that can form on the arterial wall in response to inflammation. When vulnerable plaque ruptures, blood clots can form, blocking the artery and diminishing blood flow, thus reducing oxygen supply to the heart and causing damage or death to heart muscle cells and tissues. The result is often fatal.

A wide range of factors can increase the risk of heart attack, including age, poor diet, lack of exercise, smoking, diabetes, being overweight or obese, chronic stress, high levels of physical exertion, high blood pressure, excessive alcohol consumption, the overuse of pharmaceutical or illegal drugs, kidney disease, and a personal or family history of heart disease. Risk can also be increased by various psychosocial factors, including low income or poverty, social isolation, depression, and stress. All of these factors impair survival outcomes following a heart attack.

In both men and women, symptoms of AMI may be "silent," meaning they may occur without being noticed; an estimated 25 percent or more of all cases of AMI in the United States fall into this category. When symptoms are apparent, they occur gradually, over the course of several minutes. The most common symptoms of AMI are chest pain (which can spread down the left arm and/or the left side of the neck), shortness of breath, nausea, vomiting, excessive sweating, and chest palpitations. In women, symptoms may not be as intense or as varied, and most commonly manifest as shortness of breath, fatigue, weakness, and sensations similar to indigestion. In the most serious cases, loss of consciousness or sudden death can also occur.

Because they can be fatal, heart attacks require prompt medical attention. Diagnostic tests include the electrocardiogram (EKG), which can detect abnormalities in the electrical activity of the heart that usually occur during an AMI and also identifies the areas of heart muscle that are deprived of oxygen. Various blood tests may also be used after the incident to screen for blood markers that indicate AMI has occurred.

Once a diagnosis of AMI has been confirmed, immediate treatment can include the use of oxygen, aspirin and other blood thinners (to reduce clotting), and sometimes nitroglycerin tablets (to widen narrowed blood vessels). More invasive procedures, including surgery, may also be necessary in order to unclog blocked arteries and restore the flow of blood and oxygen to the heart as quickly as possible. The more rapidly blood flow can be reestablished, the more heart muscle can be saved.

The restoration of blood flow to the heart is known as *reperfusion*. Methods of reperfusion include angioplasty and/or the placement of one or more stents inside the coronary arteries. These procedures are the preferred methods for preserving heart muscle, particularly if they can be performed within ninety minutes after AMI patients reach the hospital. If there is a delay past this time or if catheterization is not available, thrombolytics, or clot-busting drugs, may also be used. Patients with multiple blockages in their arteries may also have coronary bypass surgery in order to redirect and improve blood flow.

Following immediate care, with or without surgery, AMI patients will usually be prescribed various heart medications, which can include the continued use of aspirin, ACE inhibitors, beta blockers, blood-thinning drugs such as heparin, and/or statin drugs to control cholesterol levels and prevent a recurrence of heart attack. In addition, doctors will typically provide guidance about necessary dietary and lifestyle changes; stress management can be the key to a successful recovery.

Heart Murmur

A heart murmur is characterized by abnormal sounds heard during the heartbeat cycle. Heart murmur is not a disease, but it can be a sign of an underlying heart condition. There are two types of heart murmur: *innocent* and *abnormal.* Innocent murmurs do not require treatment and are common in cases that are present from birth, or congenital. Abnormal murmurs are more serious and can indicate inflammation in the heart, heart valve problems, or a hole in a wall within the heart's chambers. The severity of the abnormal murmur will determine the kind and intensity of its treatment.

Congenital heart murmur is linked to a family history of heart defects, or an illness and/or medication use that occurred during the pregnancy. Abnormal murmurs can appear at any time, but particularly later in life, and usually indicate a developing heart condition such as a narrow or leaky valve (see page 30). Factors that raise the risk of heart murmurs include high blood pressure, rheumatic fever, a weakened heart muscle, and a past heart attack.

People with innocent murmurs are unlikely to experience symptoms aside from the murmur itself—a disruption, extra beat, or whooshing sound that's heard when listening to the heartbeat. People with abnormal murmurs may also have symptoms that derive from the underlying condition causing the murmur, including chest pain (angina), shortness of breath, excessive sweating, dizziness or fainting, chronic cough, bluish skin (particularly around the lips and fingertips), swelling or sudden weight gain, enlarged liver or neck veins, and poor appetite and failure to grow in infants.

Physicians can detect a heart murmur using a stethoscope. The stethoscope also allows them to evaluate the murmur according to how loud it is, where in the heart it is located, when it occurs and for how long, and whether its sound changes with changes in body position. If further tests are necessary, they may include chest X-rays, an electrocardiogram (EKG), an echocardiogram, trans-esophageal echocardiogram (TEE), a CT scan, or an MRI.

Treatment is unnecessary for innocent murmurs; even with abnormal murmurs, physicians may elect to monitor the effects over time. Additional medical care, when ordered, usually treats the heart condition that is the source of the murmur, and might involve anticoagulants, diuretics, angiotensin-converting enzyme (ACE) inhibitors or angiotensin receptor blockers (ARBs), statins, beta blockers, or digoxin. If necessary, surgery or catheterization might be performed in order to repair or replace heart valves, or to patch a hole in the heart.

Heart Muscle Disease

Heart muscle disease, or cardiomyopathy, refers to any of a number of diseases that affect the heart muscle. In cardiomyopathy, the heart muscle becomes enlarged, thick, or rigid; sometimes, it is even replaced with scar tissue. As a result, the heart's ability to pump blood to the rest of the body is impaired. Left untreated, heart muscle disease can lead to heart failure and death.

There are three main types of cardiomyopathy: *dilated, hypertrophic,* and *restrictive.* Dilated cardiomyopathy is the most common of the three. In this condition, the heart's main pumping chamber, the left ventricle, becomes enlarged, or dilated, and can no longer effectively pump blood out of the heart. Hypertrophic cardiomyopathy is characterized by abnormal growth or thickening of the heart muscle, once again preventing blood from being pumped out of the heart. Restrictive cardiomyopathy is a condition in which the heart muscle weakens and loses its ability both to pump out and fill with blood between heartbeats.

Cardiomyopathy can be inherited (passed on by one or both of your parents) or acquired (developed as a result of another condition or factor). Around one-third of all cases of dilated cardiomyopathy are inherited; other risk factors include coronary heart disease or heart attack, high blood pressure, diabetes, thyroid disease, viral hepatitis, HIV, and the abuse of alcohol and certain drugs. Most cases of hypertrophic cardiomyopathy are inherited, caused by a mutation that makes the heart muscle grow especially thick; some cases, however, are associated with diabetes or thyroid disease. Restrictive cardiomyopathy is often linked to diseases such as hemochromatosis, in which excess iron builds up in your body; sarcoidosis, an inflammatory disease; amyloidosis, in which excess protein builds up in your body; and some types of cancer and cancer treatments.

In the early stages of cardiomyopathy, symptoms may not be apparent; in many cases, the first symptom will be the last—a sudden collapse due to heart failure. Otherwise, common symptoms include sensations of breathlessness, even when at rest; swelling of the ankles, feet, and legs; bloating and fluid buildup in the abdomen; fatigue; dizziness; fainting; chest pain; cough; and arrhythmia.

A variety of diagnostic tests can be used to detect heart muscle disease. Your doctor will need to take into account your personal and family history, and also screen for symptoms, including heart murmurs and swelling of the ankles, feet, abdomen, or neck veins. If cardiomyopathy is suspected, you may be asked to undergo additional tests, including chest X-rays, electrocardiogram (EKG), angiogram, MRI, or, in some cases, cardiac catheterization with biopsy, in which a catheter is inserted into the groin and then threaded upward to the heart in order to extract a small sample of heart tissue for analysis. Sometimes, your doctor will order a specific blood test that measures the level of a chemical known as brain natriuretic peptide (BNP), which is often elevated when the heart is under stress.

Treatment for heart muscle disease varies according to the type, but the primary goal is always to manage symptoms and keep them from worsening. Drugs prescribed for dilated cardiomyopathy include angiotension-converting enzyme (ACE) inhibitors or angiotensin receptor blockers (ARBs), beta blockers, diuretics, and digoxin. The insertion of an implantable cardioverter device (ICD) may also be necessary to help regulate the contractions between the heart's left and right ventricles.

Beta blockers and calcium channel blockers are the two most common classes of drugs used to manage hypertrophic cardiomyopathy. If necessary, an ICD or a regular pacemaker may be implanted. In some cases, other types of surgery may be performed. The first is known as septal myectomy, a form of open-heart surgery in which parts of the thickened, overgrown heart muscle wall (known as the septum) are removed to improve blood flow. A second type of surgery, known as septal ablation, or septal alcohol ablation, destroys a small portion of the thickened heart muscle. This is accomplished by injecting alcohol through a catheter into the artery that delivers blood to the septum.

In cases of restrictive cardiomyopathy, doctors often recommend a low-salt diet along with careful monitoring of water intake. Diuretic and blood pressure medications will often be prescribed. Beta blockers and calcium channel blockers may also be used along with blood thinners and drugs in order to regulate heart rhythm. In certain cases, a pacemaker may be surgically implanted or a heart transplant may be performed, but surgery is rarely undertaken, due to poor likelihood of success.

High Blood Pressure (Hypertension)

High blood pressure, or hypertension, affects 76.4 million Americans today. Blood pressure is essentially a measure of the force (pressure) exerted by circulating blood on the walls of your arteries. Hypertension occurs when the force becomes so strong that it begins to stretch or cause damage to the arteries. Serious cases of hypertension can eventually create other health problems, including heart attack and stroke.

There are two types of hypertension: *primary (essential) hypertension* and *secondary hypertension.* Primary hypertension usually develops gradually over many years, and can be caused by a number of genetic and environmental factors, including age, gender, race, family history, stress, excessive sodium or alcohol consumption, poor diet, lack of exercise, and being overweight or obese. Secondary hypertension is usually caused by an underlying health condition, such as kidney disease, adrenal gland tumors, congenital heart conditions, or by the use of pharmaceutical drugs, including birth control pills, cold and flu remedies, decongestants, and pain medications, and illegal drugs such as amphetamines and cocaine.

Most of the time, there are no symptoms of hypertension. When symptoms do appear, it is usually a sign that the condition has progressed and may even be life threatening. The most common symptoms are dull headaches, dizzy spells, and sometimes nose bleeds.

High blood pressure is easily diagnosed; a simple blood pressure reading can be taken using an automatic cuff-style monitor at the doctor's or even at some local drugstores. Many communities also offer free blood pressure screenings throughout the year. If you are particularly concerned, you can even buy a monitor for home use.

Usually, physicians will take two or more blood pressure readings during separate appointments before making a diagnosis of hypertension. That's because blood pressure levels vary over the course of the day, and can also spike in the presence of doctors due to nervousness or anxiety—a phenomenon known as "white coat" hypertension. For this reason, many doctors wait until their patients are relaxed and comfortable before taking blood pressure readings.

In any blood pressure reading, there are two measurements taken. The first (top) number is your systolic blood pressure, or the pressure that is exerted on your blood vessels when your heart contracts, pumping blood through your body. The second (bottom) number is your diastolic blood pressure, or the pressure exerted on your blood vessels when your heart relaxes. For people age fifty or older, a high systolic reading with a normal diastolic reading most frequently indicates hypertension. (For more information on blood pressure levels, consult the inset below.)

BLOOD PRESSURE LEVELS IN ADULTS		
CATEGORY	**SYSTOLIC (TOP NUMBER)**	**DIASTOLIC (BOTTOM NUMBER)**
Normal	Less than 120	*and* Less than 80
Prehypertension	120–139	*or* 80–90
High blood pressure		
Stage 1	140–159	*or* 90–99
Stage 2	160 or higher	*or* 100 or higher

Once a diagnosis of hypertension is made, other screening tests may be ordered to determine whether the hypertension is a symptom of an underlying condition. These include blood tests or an electrocardiogram (EKG) or echocardiogram to screen for other possible signs of heart disease, or perhaps a urine test to screen for kidney problems.

Proper treatment of hypertension begins with a healthy, low-sodium diet, regular moderate exercise, and stress management. Blood pressure medications may also be necessary and can range from diuretics and vasodilators (drugs which cause the arteries to relax and widen) to angiotensin-converting enzyme (ACE) inhibitors or angiotensin receptor blockers (ARBs), beta blockers, and calcium channel blockers. Once you have been diagnosed with high blood pressure, regular checkups will also be advised in order to monitor your condition.

Mitral Valve Prolapse

While both of the valves that connect your upper and lower heart chambers can develop disorders, mitral valve prolapse, or MVP, is the more common valve condition. In MVP, the mitral valve, which connects your left atrium and left ventricle, doesn't close properly. Instead, this valve bulges, or prolapses, into the left atrium every time that the heart muscle contracts. In some cases, this can cause blood to leak backwards into the left atrium, causing what is known as mitral valve regurgitation.

Although MVP can develop at any age, it's most common in men above the age of fifty, and tends to be inherited from a parent. A number of diseases can also increase the risk of MVP, including adult polycystic kidney disease (a genetic disorder of the kidneys), Ebstein's anomaly (a rare heart defect that causes leakage between heart chambers), or certain conditions that affect the connective tissues, including Ehlers-Danlos and Marfan syndromes. Scoliosis, or abnormal curvature of the spine, can also increase the risk of MVP.

Many people with MVP do not experience any symptoms and are therefore surprised to discover that they have this heart condition. When symptoms are present, they may include arrhythmia, dizziness, shortness of breath, fatigue, and/or chest pain. People who have MVP are at a higher risk for a condition called *endocarditis,* in which the inner tissue of the heart becomes infected with bacteria.

The easiest way to test for MVP is with a stethoscope; if MVP is present, your doctor will hear clicking sounds or a heart murmur, as both are good aural indicators of an abnormal flow of blood in the heart. Other diagnostic tests associated with leaky valve (mitral regurgitation) may include chest X-ray, electrocardiogram (EKG), echocardiogram, stress testing, and cardiac catheterization.

Most cases of MVP are not serious and do not require treatment or even changes in lifestyle. If symptoms are present, usually due to an arrhythmia or a leaky valve, your doctor may decide to monitor your condition to ensure that it doesn't worsen, or prescribe drugs such as aspirin, anticoagulants, or beta blockers. Surgery is rarely necessary, but occasionally open heart surgery is performed in order to repair or replace the leaky mitral valve.

Pericarditis and Pericardial Effusion

Pericarditis is an inflammation of the pericardium, the thin set of membranes that encases the heart. When the pericardium is inflamed, its two layers rub against each other, causing painful friction. There are two kinds of pericarditis: acute, which lasts for six weeks or less, and chronic, which can last for six months or longer. Although unpleasant, pericarditis is rarely fatal.

By contrast, pericardial effusion is more serious. In this condition, fluid builds up between the two layers of the pericardium, putting pressure on the heart and preventing it from functioning properly. Severe cases of pericardial effusion can force the heart's chambers to compress or even collapse; this condition is life-threatening and is called cardiac tamponade.

While the cause of pericarditis is not always clear, viral or bacterial infections are often to blame. Risk factors for pericarditis also include chest injury, kidney disease, heart attack, lupus, and rheumatic fever. Pericardial effusion is often, but not always, a response to pericardial inflammation. It can also be caused by viral, bacterial, fungal, or parasitic infections; autoimmune diseases (lupus, HIV); certain types of cancer; and trauma to the heart (caused by injury or surgery).

Acute pericarditis produces sharp, stabbing chest pains that come and go quickly; sufferers may believe they're experiencing heart attacks. Other symptoms include fever, weakness, difficulty breathing, and coughing. Chronic pericarditis will cause fatigue, coughing, shortness of breath, and swelling of the stomach and legs; chest pain is often absent.

Symptoms of pericardial effusion include shortness of breath or difficulty breathing, chest pain behind the breastbone or the left side of the chest that is exacerbated by inhalation and worsens when lying down, coughing, dizziness, low-grade fever, and rapid heart beat. Symptoms may not be initially apparent, manifesting only when the fluid buildup increases.

Your doctor may be able to diagnose pericarditis or pericardial effusion using a simple chest exam with a stethoscope; other tests include electrocardiogram (EKG), echocardiogram, chest X-rays, MRI, and CT scan. Blood tests may also be ordered to help determine underlying causes.

Treatment for pericarditis and pericardial effusion might include anti-inflammatory drugs such as aspirin, nonsteroidal anti-inflammatory drugs (NSAIDs), colchicine, and corticosteroids such as prednisone. If bacterial infection is suspected as the cause of the inflammation, antibiotics will be prescribed. In cases of cardiac tamponade, a procedure called pericardiocentesis or even open-heart surgery may be required in order to drain the pericardium. Often, a catheter will be left in the pericardium in order to encourage further drainage; it is then removed after a few days. Rarely, the pericardium itself will be removed, in a procedure called pericardiectomy.

Premature Ventricular Contractions

Premature ventricular contraction, or PVC, is a common condition that occurs when one of the ventricles produces an extra, abnormal heartbeat, disrupting the regular heart rhythm and thus, potentially, the flow of blood. Most people will experience a PVC at one time or another—it's often described as the sensation of the heart "skipping a beat," although in fact the heart is actually adding one.

The causes of PVC aren't always clear, but are generally thought to be rooted in faulty electrical impulses. Other factors that increase the likelihood of a PVC include biochemical changes or imbalances in the body (e.g. low potassium or magnesium), alcohol or drug abuse, overexertion, excess caffeine consumption, smoking, hypertension, anxiety, and other underlying heart conditions. Certain medications, particularly those used to treat asthma, can also trigger PVCs. While most cases of PVC are harmless, in others they can lead to arrhythmias which, if they become chaotic enough, can result in sudden cardiac death.

Many people who have a PVC will never even notice it. If you do notice, you might feel as if your heart is racing, flip-flopping, or fluttering, or as if it has either skipped a beat or stopped.

The standard method for detecting PVC is an electrocardiogram (EKG), with or without a stress test. In some cases, devices such as the Holter monitor or an event recorder can also be used. A Holter monitor is a small, portable device that can be carried in your pocket or attached to your belt. It automatically records your heart rhythms for a twenty-four hour period, so that your doctor can better detect any anomalies. An event recorder is a small portable EKG device that can also be carried on your person the way a Holter monitor can. When PVC symptoms are experienced, the recorder is activated with the push of a button so that a brief EKG recording is made. This enables doctors to see the heart rhythm as the PVCs occur.

Because PVCs are usually innocuous, treatment is rarely required for people who have no underlying heart conditions. If the symptoms are particularly frequent or troubling, however, your doctor may encourage you to make lifestyle changes that can minimize PVC triggers, such as avoiding alcohol, limiting caffeine intake, quitting smoking, and stress management. In the event that medication is required to treat a PVC, beta blockers are the drugs most commonly used.

Stroke

A stroke is caused when the blood supply to the brain is interrupted or severely reduced, either because an artery has ruptured (burst) or because it has been blocked by a clot. Deprived of oxygen and other nutrients that the blood transports, brain cells begin to die within minutes after a stroke occurs. Prompt medical attention is thus essential to limiting brain damage and other potential complications. Nearly 800,000 Americans will experience a stroke each year; it is the fourth most common cause of death in the United States and a leading cause of disability.

There are two main types of stroke. The most common is called an *ischemic stroke,* which accounts for 87 percent of all strokes each year. An ischemic stroke occurs when an artery to the brain becomes blocked by a blood clot, causing severely reduced blood flow (ischemia). There are two subcategories of ischemic strokes: *thrombotic strokes,* in which the blood clot forms in an artery that has already been narrowed (usually by atherosclerosis), and *embolic strokes,* in which the clot breaks off from another location (usually the heart) and travels to one of the brain's blood vessels, which are too narrow to allow the clot through.

Hemorrhagic stroke accounts for the other 13 percent of all strokes, and refers to a stroke that is caused by a blood vessel that ruptures and then leaks blood (hemorrhages) into the brain. There are two subcategories of hemorrhagic stroke. The first type is *intracerebral hemorrhage,* in which a blood vessel in the brain bursts, spilling its contents into surrounding brain tissue, damaging brain cells and depriving them of oxygen. The second type is *subarachnoid hemorrhage,* which is caused by the bursting of an artery or aneurysm (abnormal bulge or "balloon" in a blood vessel) on or near the surface of the brain.

A particularly acute form of subarachnoid hemorrhage is due to the rupture of an *arteriovenous malformation* (AVM). An arteriovenous malformation is an abnormal tangle of blood vessels in or on the surface of the brain; they are usually present from birth and affect less than one percent of the population. While many AVMs are harmless, they are known to hemorrhage in over half of all patients who have them, and thus must be monitored regularly.

In addition to the two main categories of stroke, you can also suffer a *transient ischemic attack* (TIA), or what is sometimes called a mini-stroke. A TIA is similar in nature to an ischemic stroke, in that it, too, is caused by a blood clot; the only difference is that in a TIA, the blood clot eventually passes through, ending the blockage. Although the symptoms are nearly identical, a TIA is not formally classified as a stroke, because the blockage is temporary, lasting five minutes or less. People who experience TIAs may suffer some brain damage, and are still at risk for a full-blown stroke later on. Because of this, prompt medical attention is recommended even when symptoms seem to be fleeting.

A variety of factors increase the risk of stroke, including poor nutrition and diet, hypertension, lack of regular physical activity, being overweight or obese, smoking or regular exposure to secondhand smoke, diabetes, a previous history of heart disease, excessive alcohol consumption, the use of illegal drugs such as cocaine and amphetamines, and sleep apnea, a condition in which oxygen levels fluctuate and drop during the night due to intermittent interrupted breathing. Use of birth control pills can also increase the risk of developing blood clots, and thus stroke. In addition, race can be a factor; statistically, African Americans have a higher risk for stroke than whites and other groups.

Symptoms vary according to the type and severity of the stroke. They include sudden dizzy spells, loss of coordination or difficulty walking, slurred speech, difficulty understanding speech, paralysis or numbness of the face, arm or leg, and blurred or blackened vision in one or both eyes. A person who suffers a hemorrhagic stroke may also experience a sudden, sharp headache, which may or may not be accompanied by vomiting. At the first sign of symptoms, dial 911 for immediate medical attention, for the sooner you receive treatment, the higher your chances will be for a successful recovery.

Ischemic stroke is more likely than hemorrhagic stroke to be fatal. In both types, the risk for a second stroke is greatest in the weeks or months following the first; thus it is vital that proper treatment and preventive measures be taken.

In order to ensure appropriate treatment, the doctor will need to identify the type of stroke suffered. A thorough physical exam will be conducted, with questions about the symptoms experienced and their duration. Blood tests will be ordered to determine more information about the levels of blood sugar and other chemicals, and to determine how quickly the body forms blood clots. The patient might also undergo a CT scan and/or MRI to detect brain damage, an ultrasound of the carotid arteries in the neck to determine blood flow and plaque build up, an angiogram of neck and brain arteries, or an echocardiogram to determine the source of blood clots in the heart.

Treatment varies according to the type of stroke suffered. For ischemic strokes, doctors focus on quickly restoring proper blood flow to the brain. This can be accomplished by giving the patient aspirin immediately following the stroke to prevent further clots from forming. Simultaneously, blood clot-dissolving drugs called thrombolytics will be administered, ideally within 4 to 5 hours after the stroke occurs; the most common thrombolytic used is called tissue plasmogen activator (TPA). In severe cases of ischemic stroke, physicians may surgically thread a thin tube (catheter) through an artery and up to the brain, in order to deliver TPA directly to the area where the stroke occurred and bust the clot. A catheter might also be used to insert a small device to mechanically capture and remove the blood clot.

In some cases, surgical measures might be taken in order to prevent the risk of a future stroke. This can be accomplished by angioplasty with stents or by a procedure called carotid endarterectomy, in which the carotid artery is opened to remove the plaque that is blocking it. The artery is then either stitched up or patched using material from another vein or an artificial graft.

In cases of hemorrhagic stroke, the focus is on controlling bleeding in the brain, and to reduce pressure caused by the bleeding. In such cases, aspirin, thrombolytic drugs and TPA cannot be given, as these drugs can cause the bleeding to worsen. Instead, drugs to lower blood pressure levels, prevent seizures, and reduce brain pressure will likely be used. It may also be necessary to repair blood vessels surgically. Procedures include surgical clipping, in which a tiny clamp is attached to the base of the damaged blood vessel or aneurysm in order to prevent it from bursting, and coiling, in which small coils are threaded into an aneurysm to block blood flow. When hemorrhagic stroke is threatened or caused or by the rupture of an arteriovenous malformation (AVM), surgery can also be performed to remove the problematic veins if they are small and easily accessible.

Treatment will also be necessary to manage the lingering after-effects of a stroke, which include loss of muscle control or paralysis on one side of the body, continued problems speaking and being understood, difficulty reading or writing, difficulty swallowing, mental confusion and memory problems, pains or numbness in the parts of the body affected by the stroke, and depression or other emotional problems. Most people require some degree of caretaking after suffering strokes, and many will need to undergo a rehabilitation program in order to regain speech and muscle capacity. A psychologist or psychiatrist may also be necessary in order to deal with any depression or other lingering emotional problems that result from the stroke. With proper treatment and rehabilitation, symptoms can improve over time, and even resolve fully.

THE RISK FACTORS

Having read about the most common types of cardiovascular disease, you now understand how serious our national epidemic is, and why it is truly "at the heart" of America's health care crisis. Although treatment options are expanding, the best way to manage heart disease is to prevent it from happening in the first place. In addition to regular screenings from your doctor, true prevention of heart disease involves addressing all of the known risk factors that increase its likelihood of occurrence. The most common risk factors for each condition were mentioned in the earlier descriptions. Now let's examine these risk factors separately in order to get a better sense of the roles they play in heart disease.

There are two categories of risk factors: uncontrollable (non-modifiable) and controllable (modifiable). As the name implies, uncontrollable risk factors are facets of your life that you have no control over, such as age, hereditary factors (your genes), a family history of heart disease, and race. African Americans, Native Americans, and Mexican Americans all have a higher risk for developing heart disease compared to whites and Asian Americans.

By contrast, controllable risk factors are those you *can* manage in order to minimize your risk of cardiovascular disease. Although doing so does not guarantee that you will never develop heart disease, at the minimum, proactive behavior allows you to improve your mindset and your health in other areas. The most common controllable risk factors are discussed here.

Being Overweight or Obese

Because of poor eating habits and a sedentary lifestyle, Americans are getting fatter. According to the CDC, nearly 34 percent of all men and women in the United States are obese (at least 20 percent over their ideal body weight), and an additional 30 percent more are unhealthily overweight, though not yet obese. Being overweight strains your heart and can contribute to other risk factors for heart disease, including high blood pressure, diabetes, and high cholesterol. If you are overweight, seek help to lose weight by eating right and exercising.

High Blood Pressure (Hypertension)

High blood pressure is the most common risk factor for heart disease, affecting nearly one in three adults in the United States. Have your blood pressure levels regularly screened by your doctor, and learn how to control it with diet, exercise, stress and/or weight management, and, if necessary, blood pressure medications. For more information, see the section on hypertension (page 28).

High LDL and Total Cholesterol Levels, Low HDL Cholesterol Levels

High levels of low-density lipoprotein (LDL or "bad") cholesterol and total cholesterol, along with low levels of healthy HDL cholesterol, have long been linked to an increased risk for heart disease. Because cholesterol is a major risk factor, your intake of this fatty substance must be controlled. Cholesterol management should be individually tailored to take into account your other specific risk factors, but will almost always involve eliminating unhealthy trans fats, junk food, and soft drinks from your diet.

Lack of Exercise

Americans live increasingly sedentary lifestyles; most of us fail to get the exercise we need. Regular physical activity will significantly reduce your risk of coronary heart disease, and provides a wealth of other benefits as well—it helps people lose weight, reduce stress, strengthen bones and muscle, and raise their HDL ("good") cholesterol levels. You don't need to be a gym rat to achieve these benefits, either. In fact, a growing body of research indicates that moderate exercise is sufficient for most people's requirements. A daily walk, gardening, bicycling, and swimming are all excellent ways to get the exercise you need. The key is to pick an activity that you enjoy doing and stick to it—getting twenty to thirty minutes of exercise each day will put you on the right path to optimal health and make you feel much better. If you are not used to physical activity, be sure to consult with your physician first before beginning an exercise program.

Poor Dental Hygiene

Historically, some studies have indicated that gum disease seemed to be associated with a higher risk for heart disease. It seemed to make good sense that bacteria from the mouth could enter the bloodstream and travel to other areas of the body—including the heart—where they would cause inflammation and contribute to atherosclerosis. More recently, however, the American Heart Association issued a statement casting doubt upon this theory. Gum disease and heart disease share certain common risk factors—including smoking, age, and diabetes—which probably account for the correlation previously observed between the two conditions. But correlation does not give us proof of causation. In other words, it is now considered highly unlikely that gum disease causes heart attack or stroke.

Even so, it is in your best interest to maintain good dental hygiene by brushing your teeth, flossing, and using a germ-killing mouthwash daily. These are all essential self-care measures you can and should take to maintain your overall health.

Poor Diet

The standard American diet is responsible for much of our nation's health care crisis, and plays a major role in many cases of heart disease. Your diet is another area over which you have a great deal of control. Emphasize foods that are healthy for you and free of chemical additives; eat an abundant supply of fresh vegetables each day, along with lean meats, poultry, and heart-healthy fish such as salmon (avoid fish that is farm-raised due to the food dyes, antibiotics, and other additives they contain), and moderate amounts of whole grains and legumes. For snacks, consider nuts or fruit in place of sweets, and avoid junk and fast food.

Smoking

Smoking is a deadly habit that affects almost every organ in your body. Tobacco is linked to one out of every five deaths in America, and is responsible for at least 30 percent of all cancer deaths. In addition, smoking is a major risk factor for cardiovascular disease. Smoking decreases the supply of oxygen to the heart, increases blood pressure and heart rate, and also causes the formation of unhealthy blood clots. Even light smoking causes damage to the heart and blood vessels, and can change the structure of blood vessels. Smoking is a major risk factor for atherosclerosis and significantly increases your risk of developing heart disease. In fact, the risk of heart attack is over 50 percent higher for smokers compared to nonsmokers, and even higher than that for heavy smokers (ten or more cigarettes a day). If you smoke, quit; seek help to do so, if necessary. If you don't smoke, but are frequently around people who do, try to limit your exposure, as people who inhale secondhand smoke also run a higher risk for developing heart disease.

Stress and Uncontrolled Emotions

Both stress and uncontrolled emotions, especially anger, significantly raise the risk for heart disease, and have been linked to higher risk for heart attack and stroke. Research has shown that chronic stress can increase the risk of heart attack by nearly 30 percent. In addition, uncontrolled stress has also been shown to elevate blood pressure and increase levels of LDL ("bad") cholesterol.

If you suffer from chronic stress or have trouble controlling your emotions, consider exploring stress and anger management techniques, either on your own or with the help of a health professional. Also consider making time for hobbies or other activities you enjoy, and for spending time with friends and family members who are supportive of your needs. By becoming more conscious of how you respond to stressful or upsetting conditions, you will start to gain better control over your reactions.

Type 2 (Adult-Onset) Diabetes and Prediabetes

Type 2 diabetes is a condition in which the blood contains high levels of unregulated glucose (sugar) due to the body's inability to produce or use a substance called insulin. If not properly treated and controlled, type 2 diabetes and its precursor, prediabetes, can cause serious damage to the heart and lead to heart attack, stroke, and other forms of heart disease. Both type 2 diabetes and prediabetes are virtually nonexistent in cultures that adhere to a healthy diet and get regular exercise, yet their incidence in the United States continues to skyrocket. Fortunately, both conditions are easily managed; with proper diet, exercise, and weight loss, prediabetes can even be reversed if caught promptly. If you suffer from either type 2 diabetes or prediabetes, be proactive and take control before your condition takes control of you.

THE MISSING LINK

As you can see, there are many aspects of your life that you can control and change in order to lower your risk for cardiovascular disease. Unfortunately, because there are many other aspects of your life that you can't control, sometimes even the best intentions go unrewarded. The fact is that many people who are overweight or have high blood pressure and high cholesterol live long lives without suffering from heart disease, while many others who have addressed these same risk factors and eliminated them are still prone to heart attacks and other heart conditions. Research shows that many patients with normal LDL ("bad") cholesterol levels still go on to develop heart disease. Although scientists today are at a loss to understand why, you needn't be.

Over the last sixty years, a tremendous body of research has accumulated on the considerable benefits of a single mineral supplement. The research increasingly indicates that this element is the missing link between all these heart conditions, a simple substance without which our bodies suffer, and which, when used as a dietary supplement, can dramatically improve your cardiovascular health, and your quality of life more generally. This substance is magnesium—and the more you know about it, the more control you'll have over your health.

The goal of this book, therefore, is to show you how vital magnesium is, especially with regard to maintaining a healthy heart and circulatory system. When taken regularly, magnesium may prove beneficial in preventing and treating the heart diseases that have so plagued our country. In the next chapters, you will see why magnesium is indeed "magnificent" and why you are almost certainly deficient in it. Then, in subsequent chapters, you will learn how the cardiovascular and circulatory systems work, the essential roles that magnesium plays in keeping them both functioning properly, what heart disease really is, what other health conditions magnesium helps to prevent and reverse, and, finally, how you can ensure that you are getting all of the magnesium you need safely and effectively.

To find out how a single nutrient can make a huge difference in your health, read on.

2

Magnificent Magnesium
and Why You Aren't Getting Enough

Living without adequate levels of magnesium is like
trying to operate a machine with the power off.
—Dr. Christiane Northrup

Without enough magnesium, cells simply don't work.
—Dr. Lawrence M. Resnick

When most people think of nutrients, they think of vitamins. Although vitamins are certainly important, by themselves they are not enough to provide your body with all that it requires to create and maintain optimal health. Equally important are the nutrients known as minerals. In this chapter, you will learn what minerals are and why they are so important to your health. Then you will read about one of the most overlooked, yet most vital minerals—magnesium—and about its many roles in the body. Finally, you will find out why so many of us today do not have enough of the magnesium our bodies need to stay healthy.

WHAT ARE MINERALS? WHAT DO THEY DO?

Minerals are inorganic elements—the nonliving matter of which our earth is composed. This means that minerals cannot be produced or synthesized in the body the way that certain vitamins can. Instead, they must be obtained through the foods we eat, or through the water we drink.

The average body is composed of approximately 60 percent water, 17 percent protein, 15 percent fat, and 3 percent nitrogen. Minerals comprise the remaining 4 to 5 percent of adult body weight, primarily concentrated in the bones, but also found in varying quantities in the body's cells, tissues, and fluids.

Minerals within the body are classified according to their weight. Minerals that make up at least 0.01 percent of total body weight are known as macrominerals, while those that account for less than that percentage are known as trace minerals or elements. Your body needs at least 100 milligrams of each macromineral every day—much more in the case of magnesium—while trace minerals are required in much smaller amounts.

Besides magnesium, macrominerals include calcium, chloride, phosphorus, potassium, silicon, sodium, and sulfur. There are ten trace minerals that are officially recognized as being necessary for optimal health. They are chromium, cobalt, copper, iodine, iron, manganese, molybdenum, selenium, vanadium, and zinc.

Minerals play many vital roles in your body, working in combination with vitamins, hormones, enzymes, and various other nutrient cofactors to regulate thousands of biological functions. Among other important processes, minerals support immune function, metabolism, blood sugar regulation, regulation of fluids, muscle contraction and relaxation, mental and cognitive function, DNA and RNA replication and repair, and cellular detoxification. Minerals are also essential for healthy cell function, helping to generate new cells to replace old ones and regulating cell permeability—that is, the capacity of a cell to receive oxygen and nutrients through the cell membrane and eliminate cellular waste. Without an adequate supply of minerals, your body could not properly produce blood, transform energy, transmit nerve impulses, maintain the integrity of its musculoskeletal system, or regulate and maintain healthy acid-alkaline balance (pH) in the blood, cells, and tissues.

Your body cannot produce minerals on its own. Therefore, it is crucial that you obtain an optimal supply of essential minerals each and every day. While in years past, this may have been achieved simply by following a healthy diet containing an abundant supply of mineral-rich foods and water, as you'll see in this chapter, food sources are no longer sufficient to provide you with all of the necessary nutrients that your body needs each day.

THE MOST IMPORTANT YET OVERLOOKED MINERAL

Now that you have a better general understanding of how important minerals are, it's time you were introduced to the most ignored yet vital mineral for your health—magnesium! Let's begin with a few facts about this amazingly versatile, powerful nutrient.

- Magnesium is named after the ancient Greek city of Magnesia, which was famed for its fertile cropland. It was later discovered that the cropland contained large deposits of magnesium carbonate, which were responsible for the highly regarded produce it yielded year after year.

- Magnesium is sometimes referred to as the "iron of the plant world," for just as iron is the primary element of the central molecule of hemoglobin, an important component of human blood, magnesium is a primary element of the central atom that makes up chlorophyll, the "blood" of plants. The only chemical difference between heme (the central molecule of hemoglobin) and chlorophyll is this primary element; the two substances are otherwise the same. This similarity is telling: Just as magnesium enables plants to convert solar energy into plant energy, so, too, does magnesium allow humans to convert plant and animal energy into human energy.

- Magnesium is the fourth most abundant mineral in the human body. Half of your body's magnesium is found in your bones, and a little less than half exists inside the cells of soft tissues like your muscles, endocrine glands, and organs, with about 1 percent of magnesium traveling freely in the bloodstream.

- Most recently, a breakthrough study reported that magnesium binding sites have been detected on 3,751 human proteins that are essential for building, repairing, and maintaining your body's cells. Binding sites are basically molecular loading docks: areas of a protein or enzyme onto which specific molecules—in this case magnesium—can attach in order to form new compounds. Without these additional molecules, the original proteins cannot be recognized and used by the body; only when magnesium binds to them can they perform the important task of regulating your body's cells. The fact that magnesium has so many binding sites indicates that magnesium's role in maintaining health and preventing disease is far greater than previously thought.

Simply put: Without magnesium, life as we know it would not exist. Yet despite magnesium's importance, over 80 percent of all Americans unknowingly suffer from chronic magnesium deficiency. And that may be a conservative estimate, since the accepted reference ranges for "normal" magnesium status have shifted over the years to reflect the already low values in the American population. As you'll see in Chapter 6, "normal" does not necessarily mean "optimal," at least where magnesium levels are concerned.

Furthermore, medical awareness of the significance of magnesium—and magnesium deficiency—continues to be low. Medical tests are only occasionally ordered to measure patients' magnesium levels. Even when they are requested, the less accurate serum magnesium test is used more frequently than the magnesium red blood cell (RBC-Mg) test. For the most part, this lack of attention is due to the relatively poor education doctors receive in nutrition, which is not considered a major focus of medical training. This is a shame. As this book will hopefully convince you through detailed scientific evidence, the many advantages conferred by magnesium merit consideration and incorporation into mainstream medical practice.

MAGNESIUM'S MANY ROLES IN YOUR BODY

Think of magnesium as the conductor of your body's biological symphony—a central figure that orchestrates the proper functioning of approximately 80 percent of the body's metabolic processes, that is, its life-sustaining actions. It does this by binding to and activating the enzymes and compounds that are responsible for more than a thousand of the chemical reactions that occur at your body's cellular level. Because magnesium is required in order to activate these enzymes and compounds, it is known as a *cofactor;* without it, your body could not carry out these vital chemical processes that allow us to function on a daily basis.

In particular, magnesium is a cofactor for a substance known as *adenosine triphosphate,* or ATP, which plays a vital role in energy metabolism—the processes by which the body breaks down proteins, carbohydrates, and fats, converting them into energy. ATP is the energy currency of the cell, the primary product made by your cell's energy factories, or mitochondria (see Chapter 4 for more information). Unless magnesium is present to activate ATP, your body simply cannot meet all of its energy needs. Simply put, ATP is essential for life, and magnesium is what brings ATP to life.

It is also a cofactor for the family of enzymes that assist in the replication and repair of deoxyribonucleic acid (DNA) and ribonucleic acid (RNA), the genetic information that tells each of your cells, tissues, and organs what they are and what they should do. Research indicates that magnesium also plays a role in stabilizing DNA and RNA.

Magnesium is required as a cofactor for vitamin C, activating one of the body's most important antioxidant nutrients for the support of the immune system. Magnesium is also a cofactor for many other nutrients, including zinc, potassium, B vitamins, copper, calcium, and vitamin D. Without magnesium, it would be difficult to absorb and use these necessary substances.

In addition, studies show that magnesium is a cofactor for certain types of hormones, and is thus integral to the regulation and maintenance of the endocrine system. In particular, magnesium activates the family of enzymes that convert cholesterol into the sex and stress hormones that are vital for our everyday life.

Magnesium has many other functions outside its capacity as a cofactor. As you'll see in Chapter 4, it plays a vital role in pro-

Magnesium Gives Us Energy!

In order to function properly, each one of your body's 100 trillion cells produces and consumes a substance called *adenosine triphosphate,* or ATP. ATP is the essential energy currency of your cells—it fuels every function that they carry out, from transmitting nerve impulses to making your muscles contract. What many people don't know is that in order for ATP to be used by the cells, it must first be joined to its primary cofactor, magnesium. Free magnesium ions bind to an ATP molecule, forming a new compound called Mg-ATP. By changing the shape and electrical charge of the original ATP, and allowing it to be more easily attracted by and dissolved into water, magnesium essentially "activates" ATP, allowing the energy inside the compound to be accessed and used by your cells. In other words, magnesium brings ATP to life! Without it, your cells simply would not be able to get the energy they need to carry out the processes that sustain us.

It's important to understand that when scientists discuss ATP as an essential energy currency, they are almost always referring to the activated, magnesium-bound compound Mg-ATP. As a matter of convenience, the Mg- prefix has simply been dropped—a decision that serves to hide the role of magnesium as the most important component of the ATP compound. Although the abbreviated notation of ATP is used more commonly than Mg-ATP in most medical and scientific texts, this book uses Mg-ATP when appropriate, in order to highlight just how important magnesium is to your body's energy.

tecting against heart disease, including heart attacks, stroke, hypertension (high blood pressure), and arrhythmias. Magnesium does this not only by ensuring proper levels of energy (ATP), but also by activating a spectrum of cardiac enzymes that help dilate blood vessels, making it easier for the heart to pump blood and more effectively transmit nutrients and oxygen to the body's cells, tissues and organs. It also helps prevent the formation of abnormal blood clots and calcium deposits in arteries and other blood vessels.

A comprehensive review published in 2012 by the *American Journal for Clinical Nutrition* brings home the importance of magnesium to heart health. The review examined previous studies involving more than 241,000 participants and found that they consistently showed an inverse relationship between magnesium intake and stroke. In other words, the less magnesium you take in, the greater your risk for stroke.

Additional research has also shown that patients with low magnesium levels have a higher risk of dying of heart disease compared with patients with higher magnesium levels. For example, researchers in Finland report that low magnesium levels suggest a greater likelihood of having a heart attack, as well as a higher rate of overall mortality.

Magnesium is also a calcium channel blocker, meaning that it prevents excess or unregulated calcium from entering the cells of the heart and blood vessel walls. Today, synthetic calcium channel blocking drugs are typically prescribed to lower high blood pressure, migraines, angina, and arrhythmia, effectively mimicking the natural job of magnesium. Magnesium can sometimes act as a natural alternative to these drugs, allowing you to improve your heart conditions without the unpleasant side effects that many of these drugs produce.

Here are some other important functions of magnesium:

- Magnesium is an essential nutrient for the proper functioning and relaxation of the body's muscles. As noted by Dr. Mildred S. Seelig, one of the world's foremost authorities on the subject, magnesium is "the mineral of motion," meaning that without it your muscles simply could not operate. Magnesium also prevents muscle cramps and spasms, and protects muscles from being injured as the result of calcium buildup.

- Magnesium also plays a key role in maintaining the structure, integrity, and proper functioning of the cell. Magnesium acts as a gatekeeper for the cell by modulating the permeability of the cell membrane, allowing ions and nutrients to enter and cellular waste products to exit. Because of its role in regulating ion exchange in nerve cells, magnesium also helps optimize nerve impulse transmission. Magnesium also helps regulate the cells' chemical reactions.

- Magnesium aids in detoxification, protecting your cells from accumulating environmental toxins, including heavy metals such as lead, aluminum, and mercury. Magnesium also acts as a cofactor in the synthesis of glutathione, a powerful antioxidant that protects against free radical damage and toxicity.

- Recent studies have shown that magnesium is an important ingredient for the production and activation of white blood cells, which are vital to carrying out your body's immune response.

- Magnesium is also essential for healthy bones and teeth. Because of its capacity as a calcium blocker, magnesium prevents unhealthy calcium buildup (calcification), particularly inside the kidneys, where it helps to prevent the formation of kidney stones made from calcium oxalate.

- Magnesium regulates blood sugar levels, helping to prevent both low and high blood sugar. Magnesium is involved in insulin production and uptake; low levels of magnesium may therefore contribute to insulin resistance, a prediabetic condition in which the body makes insulin but is unable to process it. Studies show that adults with type 2 diabetes frequently show lower-than-normal levels of magnesium on blood tests.

The list above details just a few of the reasons why magnesium is so important for maintaining optimal health in an increasingly toxic world. Unfortunately, proper magnesium intake is not always easy to accomplish. That's because magnesium, despite its great importance to your body's health and functioning, is no longer as abundant in our diet as it once was. Moreover, the magnesium that is stored in your body can very easily be drained away. This inability to obtain and retain this vital nutrient explains why so many people today are magnesium deficient. Let's take a closer look at how this problem has come to exist.

MAGNESIUM DEFICIENCY AND STRESS

More than eight out of ten Americans are deficient in magnesium. The following section will discuss some of the reasons for this deficiency. By understanding the factors that contribute to magnesium deficiency, you can take steps to minimize their impact on your health.

The single most important factor underlying magnesium deficiency is stress. Stress depletes your body of magnesium; subsequently, magnesium deficiency causes cellular energy loss, which in turn causes disease. By this daisy chain of effects, stress essentially causes disease. This is a matter of great concern, considering the prevalence of chronic stress in society today. In order to understand its effects on magnesium status and general health, let's take a closer look at the stress response.

All of us experience stress to some degree or another on a daily basis. When we do, our bodies release stress hormones, including epinephrine (adrenaline), cortisol, and aldosterone, in order to manage the tough situations we find ourselves in. The release of stress hormones is part of a basic survival mechanism that allowed our ancient ancestors to react quickly in order to protect themselves from a perceived threat. Confronted with danger (such as the approach of a sabre-toothed tiger), these hormones furnished our ancestors with a temporary burst of energy and enhanced cardiac and musculoskeletal performance, so that they could either combat the threat or escape it. Accordingly, this biochemical reaction is known as the "fight-or-flight" response. Once the danger passed, the hormones dissipated and life went on as before.

The "fight-or-flight" response is thus a built-in part of our bodies' evolutionary design, triggered not just by acute or short-term episodes of perceived danger, but by any situation we interpret as stressful. Today, most sources of stress are chronic, or long-term—attributed less to physical threats and more to unresolved social, emotional, or psychological issues. Whether you are angry, depressed, or being chased down the street by a robber, however, your body's chemical and physiological response remains the same.

Chronic stress results in a continuous release of stress hormones. These stress hormones sap your body of the nutrients it needs—most importantly, magnesium. This is because magnesium effectively buffers your stress hormones, controlling and limiting their damage. As a result, every time stress hormones are released, they draw upon and deplete your magnesium stores, thereby making it impossible for your body to carry out the thousands of vital tasks in which this important mineral plays a role.

Although chronic stress often comes in the form of social or psychological strain, stress can also develop from a variety of different sources that we might not consciously recognize. Environment and other external or chemical stimuli can act as stressors, placing your body under assault and depriving it of the nutrients it needs—including magnesium. The following is a review of some of the daily stressors that contribute to the habitual loss of magnesium. Awareness of these stressors can enable you to make better choices to avoid, or at least mitigate, their effects.

Our Devitalized Food Supply

Compared with food that was grown fifty years ago, food today—even food that is grown organically—contains greatly reduced levels of vital nutrients, particularly the minerals that your body needs. Due to commercial farming methods, farmland all across our nation has become devitalized. Modern-day farming methods have severely depleted our soil's mineral content in a variety of ways: by abandoning the centuries-old practices of spreading rock dust, forgoing the rotation of crops from season to season, and dumping tons of chemical fertilizers, pesticides, and other substances into the soil to boost production. What's more, by the time fruits and vegetables reach the marketplace, they are usually laced with preservatives and other synthetic additives. This means that while today's fruits, vegetables, nuts, and seeds may look appetizing, they lack the nutrients they once had, and instead carry with them many toxins that can actually harm you.

According to John B. Marler and Jeanne R. Wallin, researchers at the Nutrition Security Institute in Washington, D.C., this mineral depletion of our cropland is the primary cause for the decline in the nutritional value of American foods. Because of topsoil erosion and other effects of poor farming practices, American cropland has been depleted of 85 percent of its mineral content, as compared with soil from a century earlier. As the authors state in their paper, "Without minerals, soil loses the ability to support the growth of nutritious food. Soils without minerals cannot produce plants with minerals. Foods grown on soils depleted of minerals do not contain the minerals needed to maintain human health."

Marler and Wallin's findings were supported by researchers at the University of Texas at Austin, who investigated the effects of modern farming methods on the nutritional values of over forty vegetables, along with melons and strawberries. By comparing data of the crops grown in 1950 with data of the same crops grown in 1999, they found that overall the nutrient content of the 1950s foods were as much as 38 percent higher than that of the 1999 crops. Overall, the mineral content of American farmland is estimated to be one-sixth of what it was in the 1950s, the decline effected almost entirely by commercial farming methods. And this problem is further compounded by the commercial methods used to transport and store foods across our nation.

The decline in food's nutritional content is not only due to the poor quality of our soil. Other factors play a role in leaching out nutrients from our food supply, especially the development of new cultivars (plants cultivated by selective breeding). These new cultivars often sacrifice quality for quantity. That is to say that although these newer cultivars are bred to be more productive in terms of their yield—generating more plants per dollar for the farmer—they increasingly lack the ability to draw nutrients out of the soil, resulting in fewer health benefits per plant for the consumer.

The important point to remember about this is: Depleted mineral supplies in cropland means reduced levels of all nutrients in the crops that are grown on that land.

The trend toward nutrient depletion extends to our nation's commercial meat, poultry, fish, and dairy industries. Unhealthy chemicals are involved at every stage of the production processes in these industries. Early on, the animals from which our food products are derived are given injections of growth hormones to make them grow bigger, faster; they're also given antibiotics to counteract the very unsanitary conditions in which the animals are raised. Antibiotics are used in a similar fashion in the farmed fish industry, pumped into the water in which the fish are forced to circulate, along with food dyes to confer the proper color. Once the fish and animals are slaughtered, the foods produced are often irradiated.

In addition, despite industry claims, a growing body of research now indicates that genetically modified (GM) foods contain far lower concentrations of nutrients than non-GM foods. For example, as seen in the documentary film *Genetic Roulette*, the widespread use of the herbicide Roundup actually prevents plants from absorbing magnesium and other vital nutrients as they grow. Roundup is typically used in commercial farming on crops that have been genetically engineered to be "Roundup-ready," meaning that they are resistant to Roundup's active ingredient (glyphosate) and cannot be killed by it (unlike the weeds and other plants that are Roundup's target).

Not only does this practice substantially decrease the nutrient content of the plants harvested, but because high residues of glyphosate remain on the surface of the plants, these foods are also potentially toxic. GM corn, for example, has been found to contain glyphosate in concentrations nearly twenty times—that is, 2,000 percent—the level considered safe by Environmental Protection Agency. This is significant because, according to the research of Don M. Huber, emeritus professor of plant pathology at Purdue University, concentrations of glyphosate higher than 40 percent of the "safe level" have been shown to cause organ damage in animals.

Fortunately, there is a growing trend towards organic farming and healthier methods for producing meats, poultry, fish and dairy foods. But we still have a long way to go before we can expect to have foods available to us that are as nutrient-rich as the foods to which our ancestors had access.

Poor Daily Diet

Most people realize that the standard American diet (SAD)—based around processed foods full of fats, simple carbohydrates, sugar and artificial sweeteners, and other unhealthy food additives—is a major contributing factor to our nation's escalating healthcare crisis. Such a diet is not only greatly deficient in vital nutrients, but also forces your body to use up what nutrients it still has in order to assimilate and detoxify these food-like substances!

The failings of the standard American diet are borne out by government surveys, which continue to show growing nutrient deficiencies, including magnesium and other minerals, within the American populace. Studies conducted by the National Institutes of Health (NIH), for example, reveal that the vast majority of people, not only in the United States, but in other affluent Western nations as well, fail to meet 75 percent of the dietary reference intakes (DRIs) for many essential minerals. Despite this data, the need for a daily mineral intake that is adequate for optimal health continues to be overlooked, not only by the general public, but by many healthcare professionals.

What are the culprits in magnesium depletion? Food processing is a particularly significant magnesium thief. Processed food comprises not only "fast" and "junk" foods, but even certain treatments of grains, vegetables, fats and oils. This fact was made known in 1982 by Finnish researcher Heljä Pitkänen, who warned that the industrial processing of these food groups resulted in magnesium deficiency. The refining of wheat, for example, removes the "germ," or the embryo of the grain, which contains most of its essential nutrients. Without the fatty germ, wheat stays fresher and whiter for longer periods of time. This is good for the businesses that produce and sell flour with refined wheat, but not so good for the people who eat it. It is estimated that up to 82 percent of wheat's magnesium is lost in the refining process, bringing the nutritional value of refined wheat down to nearly nothing when one considers the low level of minerals the wheat started out with due to the vacuous nature of the soil.

Various popular beverages can also deplete magnesium levels. Among the biggest "beverage bandits" is soda, due to its phosphoric acid content, and commercial sports drinks, due to the high-fructose corn syrup and other additives they contain. These beverages should be avoided at all costs. Alcohol, coffee, and other caffeinated drinks also affect your body's magnesium stores because of their diuretic effects. In addition, alcohol interferes with the ability of magnesium to be absorbed in the gastrointestinal tract and causes significant magnesium loss in the kidneys. While studies show that there are health benefits to drinking wine and coffee, the key is to do so in moderation—no more than one or two glasses of beer or wine and two eight-ounce cups of coffee per day. When you do consume such drinks, be sure to increase your intake of magnesium through daily supplementation.

The lack of healthy fats is another significant factor. Contrary to popular belief, your body needs a regular supply of healthy fats, including animal fats, in order to be healthy and generate energy. Without sufficient levels of these fats, your body will most likely lack vitamin A, an essential vitamin that plays many important roles in the body and is necessary for the efficient uptake, transport, and use of minerals, especially magnesium.

Low- and high-protein diets pose other challenges. These trendy diets place added demands on the body's magnesium stores. People who take in too little protein (less than 30 grams each day) have been shown to have a reduced ability to absorb magnesium; people who take in too much risk having their magnesium stores excreted and depleted.

Similarly, following a diet based around foods that are acid-forming—including meats, poultry, fish, starches, sugars, and simple carbohydrates—also depletes your body's magnesium stores, since magnesium is one of the primary minerals your body uses to neutralize excess acid and prevent pH imbalance. The standard American diet is the epitome of a highly acidifying and unhealthy diet; thus it is no wonder that so many of us have magnesium deficiencies.

Poor Food Absorption
and Food Preparation Methods

You might think that you could get enough magnesium just by moving away from the standard American diet, adding more magnesium-rich foods to your diet, and eating them more regularly. Unfortunately, it's not that simple.

For one thing, many of the nutrients in our foods are not bioavailable; that is, these nutrients can't be properly absorbed and used by our bodies. This is particularly true of magnesium. Research shows that the human digestive system is only capable of absorbing between 35 to 40 percent of this important mineral when it is consumed; the rest of the magnesium is not absorbed, and is instead eliminated when you go to the bathroom.

Nor is bioavailability the only issue. Research also shows that most people suffer from some level of impaired digestion due to various factors such as enzyme deficiencies, a lack of sufficient stomach acid, insufficient diversity of healthy gut flora, food allergies, or other gastrointestinal conditions. These factors further diminish your body's ability to completely absorb and use the magnesium and other nutrients it obtains from the foods you eat.

Other dietary factors can also significantly reduce the volume of magnesium you obtain from your diet, even when you make it a point to eat well. Many people mistakenly overcook their food, a practice that leaches out vitamins and minerals, including magnesium. To best preserve their nutrient content, lightly steam or broil vegetables, or simmer them in water—taking care to drink the resulting broth, which will contain any nutrients drained from the vegetables. Also, try to eat at least one portion of your vegetables uncooked.

There are also many foods that are rich in magnesium, but also contain other chemical substances that inhibit its absorption. Two of the most troublesome are the classes of compounds known as *phytates* and *oxalates*. Both of these compounds occur naturally in many vegetables, nuts, grains, and legumes (beans). Phytates bind up with magnesium and other mineral nutrients, preventing them from being absorbed and forming toxic substances during this binding process. This can cause health problems and deplete your energy levels as your body is forced to divert some of its resources to eliminating the toxins formed. Soaking grains and legumes overnight minimizes the harmful effects phytates can cause.

Oxalates also bind to magnesium and prevent it from being used by our bodies. In addition, oxalate deposits can build up in the kidneys, causing kidney stones, kidney infection, and other problems. Accordingly, people who are prone to kidney stones are often advised to avoid or minimize eating foods high in oxalates, including spinach, Swiss chard, beet greens, and collard greens, as well as quinoa, cocoa and dark chocolate—all foods that are also good sources of magnesium.

Thus even with the best of intentions, a diet seemingly rich in nutrients is simply not sufficient for getting your daily dose of magnesium. This is not to say that you should give up on eating healthy foods—far from it! You should continue to give your body a fighting chance by supplying it with a well-balanced diet of organic, nonprocessed foods. Any amount of magnesium helps. As you will read in Chapter 4, by following an appropriate diet and supplementation regimen, you can easily rectify any magnesium deficiency.

Calcium and Vitamin D Supplements

Of all the magnesium thieves, calcium and vitamin D supplements are perhaps the most surprising. While it is certainly true that both calcium and vitamin D are important for optimal health, the method and quantity of your intake of these vitamins exert significant influence on your body's uptake and use of magnesium. You'll recall that magnesium is a cofactor for both calcium and vitamin D, meaning that it is required in order to activate the benefits of these substances. As you take in calcium or vitamin D, free magnesium binds to these nutrients and is thus lost for other metabolic uses.

The benefits of calcium are well known; among other advantages, it is essential for bone health. For years, doctors and nutritionists have emphasized calcium at the expense of magnesium, recommending that calcium intake be twice as much as that of magnesium (a 2:1 ratio). Now we know better. Excessive use of supplemental calcium blocks magnesium from being absorbed and thus renders it useless, while excess magnesium actually enhances the absorption and storage of calcium. The ideal ratio between calcium and magnesium should be 1:1, just as it is in most vegetables, seeds, and nuts—the food groups that are richest in these minerals. Additionally, unlike magnesium, calcium requirements can be met almost entirely through dietary sources.

In recent years there has also been an explosion of news stories touting the many benefits of Vitamin D—it encourages calcium absorption (at the expense of magnesium absorption), promotes and regulates bone growth, reduces inflammation, and boosts the immune system. Because exposure to sunlight allows our bodies to produce all of the vitamin D we need, in theory, we would not need these supplements as long as we spend adequate time outdoors—fifteen or twenty minutes each day is all that is required for most people.

Regrettably, there are several problems that make it difficult or impractical to produce vitamin D from sun exposure alone. For one thing, our busy lifestyles often prevent us from getting access to the sun. When we do go outside, we are likely to put on sunblock, which protects us against the risk of skin cancer but can prevent us from receiving the UVB rays that are needed to produce vitamin D. If you do choose to meet your vitamin D requirements through sun exposure, avoid putting on sunblock until fifteen or twenty minutes after you've been outside, and try not to wash exposed body parts with soap after sun exposure—it can take up to forty-eight hours for vitamin D to be produced in your skin and absorbed into your bloodstream.

Because of this inconvenience, alternative methods of vitamin D intake are often suggested. Many doctors currently recommend that their patients supplement their diets with synthetic forms of vitamin D at daily dosages of 1,000 International Units (IU) or higher. But other forms are available. Long before synthetic vitamin D became a hot topic in the media, many doctors advised their patients to take a tablespoon of fermented cod liver oil, a particularly rich source of food-based vitamin D.

That said, vitamin D in any form can interfere with the uptake of magnesium in the body. Magnesium is the primary cofactor involved in the production of vitamin D, which means that vitamin D cannot even be made unless magnesium is present. The more vitamin D you take, the more magnesium your body must use in order keep the vitamin D activated, depleting critical magnesium stores.

With this in mind, doctors often recommend adding magnesium supplements if you are already taking vitamin D pills. There is no reason to suspend your vitamin D intake, although it may make sense to have your vitamin D levels checked by a doctor to ensure that you are not getting too much and thus depleting your magnesium stores.

Caloric Restriction

More than half of all Americans today struggle with obesity and other weight issues. As a result, we tend to be a society of dieters. The foundation of most diet plans is calorie reduction. Most popular weight-loss diets typically advise women to reduce their total daily caloric intake to no more than 1,500 calories—500 calories less than the amount recommended by the United States Department of Agriculture (USDA)—and men to confine theirs to 1,800 calories or less—800 short of the USDA's recommendation.

While reducing caloric intake can help shed unwanted pounds, these kinds of diets can also reduce the amount of essential nutrients, including magnesium, that your body needs to achieve optimal health. When you account for the various other factors that diminish the nutrients contained in food, including those outlined above, it becomes increasingly unlikely that dieters are obtaining all of the nutrients they need. Additionally, caloric restriction puts the body under enormous stress, accelerating the rate at which you burn magnesium and thus depleting your stores of this nutrient even more quickly than usual.

If you need to lose weight, don't just cut calories; instead, make a conscious effort to eat better. Eliminate junk and processed foods, along with white flour and other simple carbohydrates, and limit your intake of other starchy carbohydrates such as breads and pasta. Instead, focus on eating moderate amounts of whole grains and legumes, along with plenty of fresh vegetables, and moderate amounts of protein foods. Also avoid high-calorie beverages, including sports drinks, commercial fruit juices, and alcohol. If you need additional help losing excess weight, consult with your doctor, nutritionist, or trainer.

As this chapter has shown, conscientiously following a healthy diet is not in itself enough to ensure proper nutrient absorption. It is, however, an important step to take in the ongoing process of optimizing your health.

Pharmaceutical Drugs

Many pharmaceutical drugs can seriously deplete the body's magnesium stores. One common culprit is proton pump inhibitors (PPIs)—including Nexium, Prilosec, Prevacid, Protonix, and Aciphex—which are frequently prescribed to reduce the stomach acid implicated in gastroesophageal reflux disease (GERD). Long-term use of a proton pump inhibitor can result in serious magnesium deficiency. Accordingly, people who take PPIs for a year or more are advised to have their magnesium levels checked by a doctor; magnesium supplementation will almost definitely be warranted.

In addition to PPIs, many other types of drugs drain magnesium from the body. Suzy Cohen, who is known as "America's Most Trusted Pharmacist," has identified the following drug classes that deplete magnesium:

Acid Blockers: Besides the proton pump inhibitors listed above, this class of drugs includes cimetidine (Tagamet), famotidine (Pepcid and Pepcid Complete), nizatidine (Axid), and ranitidine (Zantac).

Antacids: Commonly used antacids include aluminum and magnesium hydroxide (Maalox, Mylanta), aluminum carbonate gel (Basaljel), aluminum hydroxide (Amphojel, AlternaGEL), and calcium carbonate (Tums, Titralac, Rolaids).

Antibiotics: Drugs in the class include amoxicillin (Amoxil), azithromycin (Z-Pak), cefaclor (Ceclor), cefdinir (Omnicef), cephalexin (Keflex), ciprofloxacin (Cipro), clarithromycin (Biaxin), doxycycline (Doryx), erythromycin (E.E.S.), levofloxacin (Levaquin), minocycline (Minocin), sulfamethoxazole and trimethoprim (Bactrim, Septra), and tetracycline (Sumycin).

Antiviral Agents: Commonly prescribed antiviral drugs include delavirdine (Rescriptor), foscarnet (Foscavir), lamivudine (Epivir), nevirapine (Viramune), zidovudine/AZT (Retrovir), and zidovudine and lamivudine (Combivir).

Blood Pressure Drugs: Blood pressure medications include hydralazine (Apresoline); ACE inhibitors such as enalapril and HCTZ (Vaseretic); angiotensin II receptor blockers such as valsartan and HCTZ (Diovan HCT); diuretics such as bumetanide (Bumex), etacrynic acid (Edecrin), furosemide (Lasix), and torsemide (Demadex), digoxin, and any combination drug that contains HCTZ (hydrochlorothiazide).

Central Nervous System (CNS) Stimulants: The main drug is this class is methylphenidate (Metadate, Ritalin).

Cholesterol Drugs: cholestyramine (Questran) and colestipol (Colestid) are two drugs to pay attention to in this class.

Corticosteroids: Commonly prescribed corticosteroids include betamethasone (Diprolene, Luxiq), dexamethasone (Decadron), hydrocortisone (Cortef) methylprednisolone (Medrol), mometasone (Elocon), prednisolone (Pediapred Liquid), prednisone (Deltasone, Liquid Pred, Sterapred), and triamcinolone (Aristocort cream). Inhaled corticosteroids also deplete magnesium and include flunisolide (Nasarel, Nasalide), futicasone (Flonase), and triamcinolone (Azmacort inhaler).

Immunosuppressant drugs: Drugs in this class include cyclosporine (Sandimmune, Neoral) and tacrolimus (Prograf).

Nonsteroidal Aromatase Inhibitors: Drugs in this class are used to treat breast cancer in women who have entered menopause. They include anastrozole (Arimidex), exemestane (Aromasin), and letrozole (Femara).

Oral Contraceptives and Hormone Replacement Therapy Drugs: Drugs in these classes include diethylstilbestrol (DES), estradiol (Activella, Climara, Combipatch, Estrace, Estraderm, Estring, EstroGel, Femring, Menostar, etc.), conjugated estrogens Premphase, Prempro), esterified estrogens (Estratab), estropipate (Ogen), and ethinyl estradiol and levonorgestrel, both of which are found in many birth control pills.

Osteoporosis Medications: Drugs in this class are used to treat and prevent osteoporosis and include alendronic acid (Fosamax), ibandronic acid (Boniva) and raloxifene (Evista).

Selective Estrogen Receptor Modulators (SERMs): SERMS are another class of drugs used to treat breast cancer in both pre-menopausal and menopausal women. The drugs in this class are raloxifene (Evista), tamoxifen (Nolvadex), and toremifene (Fareston).

Sulfonamides: Drugs in this class include sulfa antibiotics, such as sulfacetamide (Klaron, Ovace), sulfadiazine (Silvadene), sulfa-doxine (Fansidar), sulfamethoxazole (Bactrim, Septra, Sulfatrim), and sulfisomidine (Elkosin), and certain diabetic medications, such as acetohexamide (Dymelor), carbutamide (Glucidoral), chlorpropamide (Diabinese), glibenclamide (DiaBeta, Glynase, Micronase), and tolazamide (Tolinase).

If you are on any of the above medications, or have used them in the recent past, it is likely that your magnesium levels have been negatively affected. Take a blood test to determine your magnesium status, and then supplement as needed.

Diarrhea and Other Gastrointestinal Problems

Chronic diarrhea and other gastrointestinal complaints, such as vomiting, poor absorption, overreliance on laxatives, inflammatory bowel disease, and celiac disease, can cause a significant loss of all nutrients, including magnesium. Ironically, such conditions are often due, at least in part, to magnesium deficiencies. That's because lack of magnesium can contribute to leaky gut syndrome, a condition in which unhealthy bacteria and waste matter that belongs in the intestines until the body can eliminate it passes through the gastrointestinal (GI) tract into the bloodstream, to cause a variety of health problems.

Magnesium helps to prevent and reverse leaky gut syndrome by reducing the permeability of the intestinal walls so that the contents of the GI tract stay where they belong. If you suffer from chronic GI problems, be sure to see your doctor, and increase your magnesium intake as needed.

Sweating

If you regularly engage in exercise or other physical activities, you are losing magnesium, along with potassium, sodium, and other minerals, through your sweat. Basketball fans may remember game four of the 2012 NBA Finals, during which Miami Heat superstar LeBron James collapsed to the floor and had to be helped off the court. At first, it was feared that LeBron had injured himself, but it turned out he was suffering from severe leg cramps. Leg cramps are often caused by the loss of electrolytes—that is, minerals in the blood that carry an electric charge—of which magnesium is a particularly important member.

LeBron was lucky; he was able to return to the court before the game ended. Not so lucky are the runners who suddenly die every year while engaged in training or races. Severe dehydration can cause mineral and electrolyte depletion, leading to arrhythmias that can produce fatal heart attacks.

For this reason, I recommend taking a "full-court press" of magnesium supplements on a daily basis, particularly before and after any sort of physical activity. While you exercise, don't replenish your electrolytes with a commercial sports drink; instead, use mineral-rich coconut water, or add some mineral drops to pure, filtered water.

COMMON WARNING SIGNS OF MAGNESIUM DEFICIENCY

Although magnesium deficiency is increasingly prevalent today, it often goes undetected until more serious health problems arise. Fortunately, your body can provide you with clues as to whether you need more magnesium. The following is a list of possible warning signs:

- Back and/or neck pain
- Impaired coordination
- Involuntary eye movements
- Muscle cramps
- Muscle spasms

- Muscle tension or weakness
- Muscle tremors
- Palpitations
- Tics
- Vertigo (dizziness)

Fatigue or low energy can also be another common sign of magnesium deficiency. As explained above, magnesium plays a central role in your body's ability to produce and use energy. Magnesium is also needed by your body to metabolize carbohydrates and fats, two primary food groups for energy production in the body. People with low magnesium levels will see a decline in their energy levels, becoming more easily fatigued than people who have adequate magnesium levels.

If you lack magnesium, you may also suffer from migraine, cluster, and tension headaches, particularly if they are frequent and other causes have been ruled out. Approximately 70 percent of all tension headaches are due to muscle tension caused, at least in part, by magnesium deficiency. Studies have shown that lack of magnesium plays a role in both cluster headaches and migraine.

Insomnia or difficulty staying asleep during the night is another possible sign of magnesium deficiency. Other warning signs include feelings of anxiety or irritability, hyperactivity, memory problems and impaired cognitive function, menstrual cramps and premenstrual syndrome (PMS), and unexplained respiratory problems, especially asthma.

Exaggerated responses to external stimuli can also be an indication of low magnesium. Such responses include a heightened intolerance to noise or the sensation that light is too bright. Feelings of nervousness in response to these stimuli, or being "on edge," are other possible reactions and early warning signs.

Finally, and most importantly, low magnesium levels can cause high blood pressure or trigger signs of other possible heart conditions. Early warning signs in this category include chest pain or pressure, irregular heart rate, or a racing heartbeat. If you experience any of these symptoms, seek prompt medical attention.

Because many doctors today do not screen their patients for magnesium deficiency, knowing and paying attention to these early warning signs can help you become aware of your body's need for more magnesium before its deficiency progresses and causes more serious health problems.

CONCLUSION

Hopefully, the information in this chapter has revealed just how important magnesium is to your health, and also how easily it can be drained from your body by a wide variety of stressors. Now that you are aware of the early warning signs of magnesium depletion, you will be able to determine when to increase your intake of magnesium. In Chapter 6, you will learn how to begin and maintain a magnesium supplementation program, and detail the very few risks associated with this marvelous mineral. First, however, let's explore how your heart and circulatory system actually work. By establishing a strong foundation for understanding cardiovascular disease, you will be better equipped to appreciate the many advantages of using magnesium in the fight against America's greatest epidemic.

3

Meet Your Heart

Above all else, guard your heart, for it affects
everything you do.
PROVERBS 4:23

In this chapter, you will be introduced to the most important organ in your body—your heart.

Your heart is the centerpiece of the cardiovascular system, the traffic director at the hub of a vast network of blood vessels that serves as the highway for the transport and exchange of oxygen, nutrients, hormones, antibodies, and waste products. Governed by a complex electrical system, the heart pumps blood to all areas of your body, making it possible for you to receive the ingredients you need to lead a healthy life.

To provide context for this miraculous organ, this chapter first describes the function and components of the cardiovascular system. Then it delves into a more detailed discussion of the heart, explaining how it circulates blood and how that circulation is regulated by a special electrical system. Finally, you will get a closer look at the biochemical workings of the cells that comprise the heart itself.

By obtaining a solid foundation of knowledge about the heart and cardiovascular system, you will be better equipped to understand both what happens when something goes wrong within that system (as with the heart conditions discussed in Chapter 1) and how magnesium is thus essential for the proper support of it.

THE CARDIOVASCULAR SYSTEM

Also known as the circulatory system, the cardiovascular system works to pump blood throughout your body, providing it with the oxygen and nutrients it needs in order to function properly, while simultaneously removing waste products such as carbon dioxide. The cardiovascular system has three components: blood, blood vessels (including veins, arteries, and capillaries), and the heart. Each component will be explored separately here.

Blood

Blood is a fluid whose primary function is to transport all the essential substances that your body needs in order to operate. Your body contains about four to six liters (five to six quarts) of blood, which must be constantly circulated throughout your system in order to maintain proper functioning. Most of your blood cells are made by your bone marrow, the soft, spongy material at the center of your bones; bone marrow continuously replenishes each type of blood cells, as each type of cell has a lifespan ranging from 10 to 120 days.

Blood is made up of four basic ingredients: *plasma, red blood cells, white blood cells,* and *platelets.* Plasma accounts for 55 percent of your blood; it is a yellowish, watery substance in which all the other blood cells are suspended. Although plasma is mostly understood as a medium of transport for these other blood cells, it also serves to convey *electrolytes*—dissolved salts and minerals, including calcium, sodium, potassium, and magnesium. As you'll see later on in this chapter, these electrolytes will prove significant for the proper functioning of your heart and for your body at large.

Red blood cells form the bulk of plasma's cargo, making up 40 to 45 percent of your blood's volume. Red blood cells carry out the most important task of any blood cell: distributing oxygen to your body. Without oxygen, your organs would quickly cease to work; your body would shut down and death would ensue in minutes. Each red blood cell is biconcave—shaped somewhat like a dough-nut, with a flattened center surrounded by raised sides—and quite flexible, capable of twisting and turning itself in order to squeeze through the narrowest of blood vessels. Red blood cells contain a protein called hemoglobin, which binds to oxygen and allows it to be carried throughout your system. It is from this hemoglobin that the red blood cell—and thus blood itself—gets its characteristic color.

White blood cells account for about 1 percent of your blood's volume. White blood cells defend your body from infection and invasion, either by engulfing foreign invaders and destroying them, or by producing antibodies that latch onto these invaders and disarm them. While white blood cells are integral to your immune system, an unusually high number of them can indicate the presence of a more serious infection or disease.

Finally, a very small proportion of your blood's volume is occupied by platelets. Platelets are tiny disk-shaped cells that are essential for blood clotting. They accumulate at the sites of injuries and stick together, forming a barrier between your body and the outside environment and preventing you from bleeding to death.

As you can see, blood is an indispensable substance, without which life as we know it would not be possible.

Blood Vessels

Blood is conveyed throughout your body by a network of hollow, elastic tubes called blood vessels. There are three principal types of blood vessels: *arteries, veins,* and *capillaries,* each performing a specific function.

Arteries carry oxygen-rich blood away from the heart and toward the rest of your body. All the major arteries in your body originate from the dorsal aorta, the biggest and most powerful artery of them all, which is attached to the left ventricle of the heart. After branching off from the aorta, the arteries reach out to the outer limits of your body—arms, legs, neck, and head—where they then subdivide into even smaller arteries, which in turn branch off into arteries that are even smaller still, called arterioles. From the arterioles, blood passes into the capillaries, where the oxygen, nutrient, and waste product exchange actually takes place. Because they must transport large volumes of blood and withstand high pressure from the pumping of the heart, the arteries are the widest, thickest, and most muscular of the blood vessels. In fact, arteries contribute to the pumping action initiated by the heart, using the muscles contained in the vessel walls to assist in pushing blood through your body. When you take your pulse, either by touching your wrist or along the side of your neck, you're actually feeling the throb of an artery as it expands and contracts to help propel blood to your extremities!

Veins are essentially the darker twins of arteries, their function mirroring or complementing that of the arteries. If arteries convey oxygen-rich blood away from the heart and toward the capillaries, veins provide the return trip, taking blood that has lost its oxygen and nutrients back from the capillaries and transporting it toward the heart. Just as all arteries stem from a larger artery attached to the heart (the aorta) and branch off into smaller and smaller arteries, ending in the arterioles, so too do all veins stem from two larger veins attached to the heart (the vena cavae), subdividing into smaller and smaller veins that culminate in venules. Veins are similar in structure to arteries, but because their load of deoxygenated blood exerts comparatively less pressure on the vessel walls, veins tend to be slightly thinner and less muscular than arteries. Veins are also unique in that they contain valves, which regulate the flow of blood and keep it moving toward the heart. Due to the way light is refracted through the layers of the skin, the deoxygenated blood that travels in your veins tends to look blue from the outside, although it is actually dark red.

The capillaries are the tiniest of the blood vessels—measuring only one cell wide—but their thin, highly permeable walls allow them to perform the oxygen and nutrient exchange that is the true purpose of the entire cardiovascular system. From the arterioles, the capillaries receive red blood cells containing oxygen and nutrients, which are then released through the capillary wall to the tissues surrounding them. After the tissues have finished processing the oxygen and nutrients, the capillaries then take any resultant carbon dioxide and waste products and absorb them back into the red blood cells, which then begin the return trip to the heart via the venules. For every artery, there is a vein running parallel to it; the capillaries provide a network or interface for transactions between these two larger blood vessels and the tissues they serve.

If all of your body's blood vessels were stretched out from end to end they would make a continuous chain about 60,000 miles long—that's more than twice the circumference of the earth! This fact is even more amazing when you realize that your heart moves the approximately six quarts (5.6 liters) of blood that are contained in the adult human body through this entire network an average of three times every minute of your life (once every twenty seconds). All this is made possible by an incredible powerhouse of energy—the heart.

THE HEART

Your heart is the most complex of all the organs in your body. While its primary function is to circulate blood through itself and the rest of the body, the heart also acts as an endocrine gland, producing hormones that allow it to regulate the flow of blood. Moreover, the heart is governed by an electrical system that dictates how and when to pump blood in the first place. Clearly, this is not a simple organ.

The heart is a hollow, fist-sized organ located roughly in the center of your chest, between your lungs and surrounded by your ribcage. It is composed almost entirely of *cardiac muscle.* Cardiac muscle is a special type of muscle tissue that possesses the characteristics of both of the two other main types of muscle that humans have. Like skeletal muscle, which generally controls voluntary movement (walking in a straight line, for example), cardiac muscle is *striated* (grooved). Like smooth muscle, which is associated with various internal organs, however, cardiac muscle is also considered an *involuntary* tissue, because it functions automatically, without direction from the central nervous system. Because

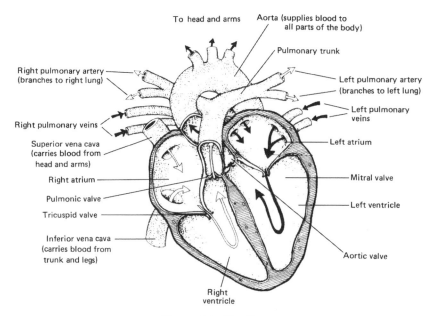

To head and arms

Aorta (supplies blood to all parts of the body)

Pulmonary trunk

Right pulmonary artery (branches to right lung)

Left pulmonary artery (branches to left lung)

Left pulmonary veins

Right pulmonary veins

Superior vena cava (carries blood from head and arms)

Left atrium

Right atrium

Mitral valve

Pulmonic valve

Left ventricle

Tricuspid valve

Inferior vena cava (carries blood from trunk and legs)

Aortic valve

Right ventricle

Figure 3.1. The Heart

it is both striated and involuntary, cardiac muscle is incredibly durable and self-regulating—uniquely qualified to keep pumping hour after hour, day after day, year after year.

The heart is encased in a thin yet tough sac called the *peri-cardium*. Filled with fluid, the pericardium's job is to protect the rest of the heart from trauma and friction from surrounding organs and structures. The heart itself is made up of three layers of muscle tissue: the *epicardium* on the outside wall, the *endocardium* on the inside of the heart cavity, and the thickest layer of heart muscle, the *myocardium,* between them.

The heart has four chambers: two *atria* (left and right) on top, and two *ventricles* (left and right) on the bottom. Generally speaking, the atria receive blood and the ventricles discharge it. The heart is further subdivided: The left side of your heart is separated from the right side of your heart by a muscle wall called the septum. Each side uses a special valve to help channel blood between its respective atrium and ventricle—the *tricuspid valve* regulates the flow of blood between the right atrium and right ventricle and the *mitral valve* regulates the flow of blood between the left atrium and left ventricle. In addition, there are two other valves that connect each of the two ventricles to their corresponding arteries—the *pulmonary valve* connects the right ventricle to the pulmonary arteries, and the *aortic valve* connects the left ventricle to the aorta.

When your heart beats, the "lub-DUB" sound you hear is created by the closing of these two sets of valves. During the first and longer part of the heartbeat, or *diastole,* the atria and ventricles first relax, filling with blood. After receiving a signal from the SA node, the atria contract and push blood more forcefully into the ventricles through the tricuspid and mitral valves. When the ventricles are completely filled, these valves close to prevent the blood from flowing backwards, creating the "lub" sound. During

Your Heart Is Also an Endocrine Gland

Most people know that the heart's main purpose is to pump blood throughout your body. But did you know that the heart can also produce hormones? Over the last fifty years, a growing body of research has shown that the heart acts as an endocrine gland, secreting at least three hormones: *atrial natriuretic peptide* (ANP), *brain natriuretic peptide* (BNP), and *c-type natriuretic peptide* (CNP). Among other functions, these hormones serve to lower blood pressure by maintaining electrolyte balance, dilating (widening) blood vessels, and reducing the volume of blood through them. Although the full significance of these hormones is still unclear, initial evidence indicates that they might have enormous implications for both treating and potentially preventing heart disease.

The discovery of these three hormones has revolutionized the way scientists look at the heart. No longer is the heart considered to be a simple pump; it is, in fact, a complex, powerful, self-regulating machine with many different capacities, not all of which are totally understood.

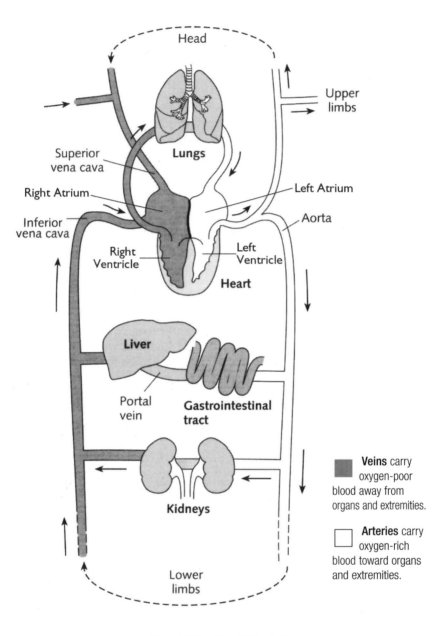

Figure 3.2. Blood Circulation

This image is a stylized representation of the ways blood circulates in the body. It is important to note that in reality, vein and artery systems overlap and interact.

the second part of the heartbeat, or *systole,* the ventricles contract, sending blood out of the heart and into the main arteries through the pulmonary and aortic valves; when these valves snap shut, we get the "DUB" sound.

Your Heart's Circulatory Function

Each side of the heart performs a distinct circulatory task. The right side is responsible for *pulmonary circulation,* or the circulation of blood to the lungs: Deoxygenated blood from all areas of the body pours into the right atrium through the vena cavae and is channeled into the right ventricle, which pumps it to the lungs in order to pick up oxygen and drop off carbon dioxide. The left side is responsible for *systemic circulation,* or the circulation of blood to the rest of the body: After the blood receives oxygen from the lungs, it returns to the left atrium of the heart via the aorta and is channeled through to the left ventricle, which pumps this new oxygen-rich blood to the rest of the body. Two of the most important destinations for this blood are the kidneys, which filter out waste products like urea and salts and excrete them through urine, and the small intestine, where the blood receives vital sugars and other nutrients released by the digestive processes.

Pulmonary and systemic circulation occur simultaneously; with every beat of the heart, blood is pushed forward on its journey through the body. At the same time, a third type of circulation is also taking place. The heart is a voracious producer and consumer of energy; in order to ensure that this hard-working muscle has the oxygen and nutrients it needs to keep pumping blood, our bodies have developed a separate circulatory circuit whose sole purpose is to feed the heart and cart away its waste products. In this process, called *coronary circulation,* special coronary (heart) arteries that stem from the aorta push oxygen-rich blood into the heart muscle (myocardium) itself. When the heart has used up the oxygen and other nutrients, the depleted blood is then rerouted by special coronary veins to the right atrium of the heart; from there it reenters the pulmonary circuit to retrieve fresh oxygen.

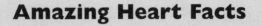

Amazing Heart Facts

- Your heart is almost entirely composed of muscle; the amount of work that it performs in a single hour is enough to lift a small car weighing approximately 3,000 pounds one foot off the ground.

- The heart beats an average of 103,000 times per day every day of your life. That equates to approximately 37.6 million times a year and 26 billion times over a seventy-year-long lifespan.

- The pressure created in your heart during a single heartbeat is enough to propel blood a distance of nearly thirty feet.

- The average volume of blood pumped per heartbeat when you are at rest is 2.5 ounces. Over the course of 24 hours, your heart thus moves nearly 2,000 gallons (approximately 20,000 pounds) of blood. That's 62,000 gallons each month and 744,000 gallons each year!

The heart is the most efficient consumer of oxygen in the body, extracting 70 to 75 percent of available oxygen from blood while other organs (such as the liver) can only obtain about 20 to 45 percent. Because the heart is so good at extracting oxygen from the blood, however, the coronary arteries tend to be fairly narrow, admitting the smallest volume of blood that the heart needs to continue working. And because the coronary arteries are so narrow, blockages to them, as in atherosclerosis, can be particularly dangerous. It is vitally important that the heart receive a continuous supply of oxygen and nutrients; when deprived of these substances, as you saw in Chapter 1, your heart—and you—will quickly die.

But how does the heart know when to beat? What keeps the heart from stopping?

Your Heart's Electrical System

Although most people understand that the heart's basic purpose is to circulate blood around the body, few people know that this circulatory function is made possible by the heart's internal electrical system, or *cardiac conduction system*. The heart's electrical system creates signals that tell the heart when and how to beat; without these electrical impulses, blood wouldn't be able to circulate at all. Thus the heart is not only a pump, but also the electrical generator that allows it to perform its pumping action in the first place. Producing signals that create their own measurable magnetic field, the heart is quite literally a source of power.

There are three parts to the heart's electrical system: the *sinoatrial (SA)* node, located in the right atrium near the entrance of the superior vena cava; the *atrioventricular (AV)* node, located on the floor of the right atrium near the right ventricle; and the *His-Purkinje system*, which consists of bunches of fibers dispersed along the ventricle walls. All three components are made up of cardiac pacemaker cells, which are specialized heart cells that are uniquely capable of generating their own electrical signals. Cardiac pacemaker cells operate automatically and independently from the body's central nervous system. Although your actual heart rate is always being adjusted by the autonomic nervous system (ANS) to meet the body's particular energy and oxygen requirements, even without any such input from the ANS, your heart's pacemaker cells can maintain a steady beat. As long as these sophisticated cells are still alive, your heart will continue to beat—even if your brain has died, and even (for a time) if your heart is taken out of your body!

Here's how the electrical system regulates the heartbeat, or *cardiac cycle*. The SA node acts as a natural pacemaker, regulating the rhythm of the heart. During diastole (see page 73), the SA node generates and sends out an electrical signal telling the atria to contract, pushing blood through the tricuspid and mitral valves and into the ventricles. The original impulse continues to travel along an electrical pathway, eventually arriving at the AV node. Once there, the signal slows briefly, allowing the right and left ventricles to fill with blood. When this is accomplished, the signal continues on to the His-Purkinje system, where it initiates systole by dispersing throughout the ventricles and stimulating them to contract, pushing blood through the pulmonary and aortic valves and out to the aorta and pulmonary artery. After the ventricles have expelled their blood, they relax, allowing new blood to enter. And then the entire cardiac cycle begins all over again, ensuring that your heart beats 60 to 100 times each minute, every minute, 24 hours a day.

For every heartbeat, therefore, there is first an electrical signal. The specific number of signals—or the number of times the heart beats each minute—depends on the amount of oxygen your cells demand. When your body requires more oxygen, say, because you're going for a run or dealing with a stressful emotional situation—sophisticated biofeedback mechanisms within your nervous system sense this need and direct the SA node to fire more frequently, causing your heart to beat faster and deliver more oxygen to your cells.

Whether your body is at work or at rest, your heart's electrical system is constantly producing signals that allow your heart to keep functioning. If the electrical signal is interrupted in any way, the result is an arrhythmia (see pages 11 to 14). The most common way to evaluate the proper functioning of your heart's electrical system remains the electrocardiogram (EKG), which measures the strength, frequency, and path of your heart's electrical signals as they travel from the top to the bottom of your heart. Increasingly, other tests are also being used, including the magnetocardiograph, which measures the strength of the magnetic fields created by your heart's electrical signals.

Now that you have a more general idea of how the heart's electrical system works, and why it is essential to proper circulation, let's delve deeper, exploring the way this system works at the cellular level.

How The Cells of Your Heart Muscle Work

Your heart muscle is made up of special cells called *cardiomyocytes* (literally "heart muscle cells"). As you have read, these cells have two essential functions. One is electrical: to conduct electrical signals initiated by the SA node. The other is mechanical: to contract and relax, helping to push blood through the cardiovascular system. Essentially, the electrical function supports the mechanical function—the electrical signals conducted by your pacemaker cells make it possible to perform the more fundamental task of pumping blood.

How do these functions take place on the cellular level? Think of your heart as a car, with each of its cells acting like a tiny rechargeable battery. In order for a battery to function properly,

What is Defibrillation?

Anyone who has ever seen a television show set in a hospital is probably familiar with the sequence of events that unfolds when a patient goes into cardiac arrest. Doctors rush in and apply two large paddles to the patient's bare chest, delivering a shock that dramatically jolts the patient back to life.

In reality, the process of defibrillation is a bit more complicated. Although on television it may look like the defibrillator uses an electrical shock to restart the heart, the opposite is true—the electrical shock actually *stops* the heart! By stunning the heart, the defibrillator effectively resets the heart's batteries, allowing the SA node to initiate a new electrical signal from a resting position.

Moreover, because they serve to reset the heart, defibrillators can be used not only to treat cardiac arrest, but also cases of severe or chronic arrhythmia, in which electrical disturbances have caused an abnormal heartbeat. Consequently, there are several different kinds of defibrillators available for use besides the manual external defibrillator you've seen on television. There are also automatic external defibrillators (AEDs), which are simpler units that use advanced computing to analyze the heart rhythms of the patient automatically before delivering the shock, and can be used by the public with little to no prior emergency care experience. For patients with chronic life-threatening arrhythmias, a special type of defibrillator called an implantable cardioverter-defibrillator (ICD) can be surgically inserted into the heart, where it can monitor the heartbeat more closely and deliver shocks as needed.

it needs a constant supply of electricity. This the heart muscle cell gets from four minerals—calcium, magnesium, sodium, and potassium. Each of these minerals carries a specific electrical charge; for this reason, they are also known as *electrolytes* or *ions*. These electrolytes exist in a state of flux within your body. Because your body is essentially homeostatic—that is, it regulates itself in order to maintain a certain physiological equilibrium—it uses a system of checks and balances to keep its electrolytes at constant, optimal levels. Thus, the presence of magnesium helps to counterbalance the presence of calcium (and vice versa), and the presence of potassium helps regulate the presence of sodium (and vice versa).

When a cardiomyocyte is at rest, calcium and sodium ions can be found on the outside of the cell, with magnesium and potassium ions on the inside. Because of the differences between

The Calcium Connection

Each of your cardiomyocytes is a rectangular cell encased by a thin membrane. This membrane is highly permeable, studded with special channels through which only specific electrolytes can pass—sodium channels for sodium ions, potassium channels for potassium ions, and so on. As you read earlier, an electrical signal, or *action potential,* is generated when ions on the outside of the cell (calcium and sodium) pass through their respective channels and switch places with ions on the inside of the cell (potassium and magnesium), creating an electrical imbalance.

But how is this action potential (electrical signal) is converted into action (muscle contraction)? The electrolyte that is the key to this process is calcium. When a cardiomyocyte receives a signal, the calcium ions are the first to respond, commanding the calcium channels in the cell membrane to open up. With the doors to the cell flung wide, calcium ions flood the interior of the cell, initiating the process by which the electrical signal is conducted, and, with ATP, enabling the chemical reactions that allow the muscle fibers in the

the specific concentrations of these electrolytes, an electrical imbalance is built up between the inside and the outside of the cell, resulting in a net electrical potential that is slightly negative. When the cardiomyocyte receives a signal from the SA node, however, the electrical imbalance is reversed: The electrolytes switch positions, with the calcium and sodium rushing into the cell and the magnesium and potassium pouring out of it. As this switch occurs, the electrical potential of the cell changes from negative to positive, creating a tiny electrical current that essentially discharges the battery and sends an electric signal down the cellular conduits of your heart.

Clearly, your heart depends on electrolytes in order to generate and conduct electrical signals. Whenever your electrolyte levels are disrupted due to either dehydration or overhydration, the functioning of your heart's electrical system is compromised, leading to arrhythmias and, occasionally, cardiac arrest. Accordingly, it

cardiomyocyte to band together and contract. As soon as the muscle fibers contract, however, magnesium re-enters the cell, forcing the calcium back out. Once the calcium ions leave the cell, the muscle fibers are no longer able to perform the chemical reactions that let the cardiomyocyte contract; as a result, the cell relaxes.

While you might think that having lots of calcium in your blood stream would be useful, the opposite is true. The more calcium ions enter the interior of your cardiomyocytes, the more frequently and forcefully your heart will contract, increasing your blood pressure and thus your risk of hypertension. In fact, special drugs called calcium channel blockers are often prescribed by doctors in order to treat hypertension or angina. By obstructing calcium's access to the interior of your heart cells, these drugs slow the rate at which your heart contracts, effectively lowering your blood pressure. But there are better ways to prevent this surplus of calcium. As you'll read in Chapter 4, magnesium regulates calcium naturally; taken in adequate doses, magnesium can actually act as a calcium channel blocker, limiting the amount of calcium that enters your cells, and thus preventing hypertension.

is essential that you have a steady supply of these important minerals; without them, your heart's batteries simply can't charge.

Once the battery is charged, your heart is primed to do the mechanical work of contracting and relaxing. But in order for this work to occur, your heart cells needs one more important ingredient—adenosine triphosphate, or ATP, the essential energy that fuels your body's cells. In the analogy presented above, if your heart is a car and electrolytes power the batteries, then ATP is the gas that lets the car move forward.

And boy, is your heart a gas-guzzler! All of your body's 100 trillion cells require ATP to function, and your cardiomyocytes are no exception. In fact, your heart muscle cells are the most voracious users of ATP—after all, it takes an enormous amount of energy to push the equivalent of 20,000 pounds of blood around your body every day! Because your heart works harder than any other organ in your body, its cells need more ATP as well. For this reason, cardiomyocytes have the body's highest concentration of mitochondria, the cellular factories that manufacture ATP. It therefore makes sense that your heart also has the highest concentration of magnesium ions in your body. This is because magnesium is essential for the biological activation of the ATP molecule. A free magnesium ion binds to an ATP molecule, changing its shape and electrical charge and forming a new compound called Mg-ATP, from which your cells can now extract the energy they need to function. Your heart thus makes and activates the greatest supply of Mg-ATP in your body—and quickly puts it to work.

Once your cardiomyocyte has access to these Mg-ATP molecules, it is finally ready to perform the contraction that the electrical signal ordered. Fueled by Mg-ATP, the heart muscle cell contracts; as soon as it does so, its electrolytes switch back to their original positions, with calcium and sodium on the outside of the cell and potassium and magnesium on the inside. The electrical signal is thus released, passing on to the next cell; accordingly, the cardiomyocyte returns to its resting state and relaxes, ready to receive the next signal. (For a more detailed explanation of the process by which the electrical signal is turned into mechanical work, see the inset on pages 80 to 81.)

CONCLUSION

Hopefully by now, you should have a clear understanding of the cardiovascular system, particularly the heart. The heart is a complex organ—it not only manages multiple circulatory functions, but also regulates this circulation through an electrical system and the secretion of its own hormones. As the hardest-working organ in your body, the heart is both a massive consumer and producer of energy, a nuclear plant that requires enormous volumes of energy in order to produce the power that keeps your body working.

As this chapter has demonstrated, minerals are integral to the two essential functions of the heart. In the form of electrolytes, they allow for the conduction of electrical impulses. And as the activator of the energy compound ATP, magnesium helps fuel muscle contractions. But what happens when your body is deprived of these important minerals? Read on! Chapter 4 will examine the consequences of magnesium loss for your heart, unveiling a new theory that raises awareness of magnesium deficiency as a potential source of cardiovascular disease.

4

The Missing Link
Magnesium Deficiency & Heart Disease

*Most modern heart disease is caused
by magnesium deficiency.*
—Dr. Mildred S. Seelig

Heart disease is the single most serious health epidemic facing the United States today. It is an enormously complex problem whose causes and risk factors the medical research community is still endeavoring to understand. Despite advances in scientific understanding, medical technology, emergency response, and health education, Americans continue to suffer heart attacks and strokes in overwhelming numbers. The statistics show that the battle against heart disease is far from over—in fact, it may just be beginning.

So what causes heart disease? Why does it occur, and why is it still such a pervasive problem? What have we failed to see? Are there factors in the development of cardiovascular disease that have not previously been considered? In short—what are we missing? It is time for some new answers to this old problem.

Chapters 1 and 3 established the foundations for understanding heart disease, introducing you to the cardiovascular system and describing the most common disease conditions affecting it. This chapter delves into the causes, risk factors, and mechanisms of heart disease. First, you will learn how the medical community presently views the development of heart disease, and how it treats and controls the perceived risk factors. Then, you will be introduced to a new theory that may account for the gaps in the system, a theory that explains why people continue to die of heart attack and stroke, despite the wealth of accepted wisdom on the subjects. The starved heart theory of heart disease proposes that there is an important and overlooked factor—a missing link—that could be the root cause of all cardiovascular disease. This missing link is magnesium deficiency, and it is implicated in every stage in the development of heart disease, from beginning to end.

By showing you that magnesium deficiency is an important and underappreciated cause of cardiovascular disease, this book will empower you to make better decisions about your treatment options, putting your well-being back into your own hands. The benefits of magnesium for heart health are no secret, yet surprisingly few people are aware of this marvelous nutrient. It's time for this to change.

THE CURRENT VIEW OF HEART DISEASE

When doctors and scientists talk about why heart disease arises, most of the time they're discussing the development of a cardio-vascular condition called atherosclerosis, in which the arteries become narrowed or hardened due to the buildup of a fatty substance called plaque. Atherosclerosis is important because it sets the stage for the development of many other serious heart conditions, including heart attack, chest pain (angina), and stroke. Find the cause of atherosclerosis, researchers reason, and you'll find the cause of many of the most common forms of heart disease.

How Does Heart Disease Develop?

Over the last twenty years, the medical community has come to believe that the root cause of atherosclerosis—and thus much heart disease—is chronic inflammation. This idea was first formally introduced in the mid-1990s by then-president of the American Heart Association Valentin Fuster and further refined a decade later by Peter Libby, the director of the Donald W.

Reynolds Cardiovascular Clinical Research Center at Harvard University. According to Fuster and Libby, inflammation is the mechanism that drives the development of both atherosclerotic (hard) plaque and vulnerable (soft) plaque—an unstable material that can easily rupture, producing clots that can block arteries and cause heart attack or stroke.

To understand Fuster and Libby's theory of how heart disease works, we first need to look at the concept of inflammation. Inflammation is essentially an immune response—your body's way of coping with an injury or threat to its well-being. There are two types of inflammation: acute and chronic. Acute (short-term) inflammation occurs in response to a bodily insult: a cut, an infection, a burn, or other physical injury. Within seconds of cutting your finger, for example, your body's immune response kicks in, sending blood cells, proteins, and other compounds to the affected area and begin the healing process. Your finger turns red, bleeds, and swells as blood rushes to the area. Eventually, the blood clots around the cut, and the redness and swelling reduces as the healing process advances. That is your body's immediate "acute inflammation" response at work.

Chronic (long-term) inflammation occurs when an acute inflammation response fails to heal or resolve an injury, or in response to prolonged exposure to a stressor. Sometimes chronic inflammation can even occur in the absence of any harmful or invasive agent. As your body tries to heal itself without success, the types of cells that are present at the site of the injury start to change, potentially causing extensive damage to both healthy and the already-impaired tissue. Because it often affects internal organs, chronic inflammation usually lacks the obvious symptoms that characterize acute inflammation, and can be difficult to diagnose. Its effects, however, are quite powerful: Because of the progressive damage it inflicts on your tissues, chronic inflammation has been linked to a number of serious health conditions, including arthritis, asthma, gastrointestinal disorders, cancer, and, of course, heart disease.

According to the inflammation model of heart disease, when an artery is torn, ruptured, or otherwise damaged by infection, high blood pressure, cigarette smoke, or other offending factors, your body initiates an inflammatory response, ordering cholesterol, blood cells, clotting proteins, minerals, and other agents to the site of the damage in order to protect and heal it. These agents embed in the wall of the artery and slowly accumulate, forming a pliable substance called soft plaque, whose outer surface is covered by a fibrous cap. Unfortunately, sometimes this cap is very thin, making the plaque unstable, easily damaged, and prone to rupture. For this reason, scientists refer to this type of plaque as vulnerable plaque.

After a time, the body begins to treat this vulnerable plaque as a new invader, essentially instigating an inflammatory cascade, or an inflammatory response to the original inflammatory response. In this new inflammatory response, fresh blood cells, cholesterol, minerals, and other healing agents are sent to fight the plaque. There are two possible outcomes to this event. When attacked by these blood cells, the fibrous cap that covers vulnerable plaque can rupture, spilling the powerful coagulants found in its interior into the bloodstream, where they thicken the blood and can form large and lethal clots. Left untreated, these clots can block the arteries—a condition called thrombosis, which ultimately leads to heart attack or stroke.

Alternatively, the calcium and other minerals sent to the plaque can help stabilize it, adhering to the plaque's sticky surface and solidifying its fibrous cap. At first glance, this inflammatory response might seem like a good thing—an attempt to protect your body against further damage—since the plaque can no longer rupture, causing thrombosis. But in fact, this outcome is still troublesome, since the plaque is now there to stay, building up in the artery walls and causing them to harden and narrow. In short, as a result of the inflammatory cascade, atherosclerosis develops—opening up new risk for a host of other cardiovascular conditions, including angina, heart attack, stroke, and more.

The discovery of vulnerable plaque has been instrumental in changing the way doctors understand heart disease. While atherosclerosis is still an important point of focus, vulnerable plaque's capacity to rupture and cause heart attacks make it potentially more dangerous than an artery blockage, no matter how extensive.

Knowing what they know, how do doctors then decide to treat heart disease?

How is Heart Disease Treated?

Because scientific understanding of inflammation is still developing, physicians in the United States treat and prevent heart disease in part by attempting to control the risk factors that seem to contribute to its development. As you'll recall from Chapter 1, some of the most commonly recognized risk factors for heart disease include smoking, poor diet, lack of exercise, being overweight or obese, stress, high blood pressure, diabetes, high LDL cholesterol or triglycerides, and low HDL cholesterol.

Many of these risk factors can be reduced or removed by adopting lifestyle changes—quitting smoking, eating a more wholesome diet, becoming more physically active, maintaining a proper weight, and eliminating or limiting stressors. In addition, doctors often prescribe drugs to help control these risk factors, including angiotensin-converting enzyme (ACE) inhibitors, angiotensin receptor blockers (ARBs), and beta blockers.

The risk factor that doctors most frequently focus on and treat through medication is high cholesterol. Although many new studies show that cholesterol is simply not the evil it is made out to be, large-scale research studies consistently identify cholesterol as one of the prime culprits in raising the likelihood of heart disease. As a result, doctors often try to lower cholesterol in their patients by prescribing a class of drugs called statins. Recommended by most major medical institutions, including the American Medical Association (AMA), the American Heart Association, the American College of Cardiology, and many others, statins are among the most widely prescribed medications in the United States. Statins do work—but not for everyone. Studies reliably show that statins either reduce or prevent the recurrence of coronary events (heart attacks, strokes, etc.) in patients who have already experienced one.

The problem is, statins are also overwhelmingly prescribed for patients who have high cholesterol levels but who have never experienced a cardiac event. In an important review of eleven of the largest-scale studies investigating the use of statins, with a combined data pool of over 65,000 subjects, a recent report published in the *Archives of Internal Medicine* found that there was no evidence that statins had any benefits for heart disease prevention in patients who had never before been diagnosed with a cardiovascular condition. While other studies have indicated limited benefits for using statins to prevent coronary events in those with no history of heart disease, much evidence suggests that if you have never had a heart attack or stroke, statins may not help you avoid them. For some, statins may even do more harm than good, as many patients suffer unpleasant side effects without definite proof of benefit.

If statins can't prevent heart disease in people who are at risk for developing it, why prescribe them so liberally? Moreover, why do people with normal cholesterol levels sometimes die of heart attacks? Is it possible that there are risk factors for heart disease that scientists have not yet considered? Or, more significantly, is it possible that there is a potential *cause* of heart disease that the medical community has overlooked—one that would allow us to formulate better treatment and prevention options by remedying the problem at the source? What is the missing link that will allow us to better understand heart disease—and prevent it?

The next section will outline an important emerging model that provides us with this missing link. The starved heart model presents compelling evidence as to a potential cause of cardiovascular disease, and proposes a simple way to both treat it and prevent it from ever developing in the first place.

THE STARVED HEART MODEL

Without food, your body begins to degenerate, and you will starve to death within thirty to sixty days. Without water, the starvation process is even quicker; you die in less than a week. The principle is straightforward: When deprived of the fuel that allows it to function, your body's vital processes begin to break down, and shortly thereafter, your body simply ceases to work, with death occurring first at the cellular level before progressing to your organ systems.

Similarly, when your heart is deprived of the energy it needs to keep blood flowing through your system, it also stops working and begins to die. Your heart needs many different ingredients to make the energy (ATP) it needs in order to function properly. If you are denied food and water, as above, you'll lack almost all the elements needed to produce ATP. But your heart can suffer and fail even when you receive seemingly adequate nutrition. Although you might not be able to see it, your heart is still starving—not for food or water, but for the most important component of ATP: magnesium. As you'll recall from Chapter 2, in order for ATP to be used by your body, it must first be bound to magnesium. Magnesium activates ATP, allowing it to perform all of its essential tasks.

Thus it is magnesium, or, rather, the lack of magnesium, that forms the foundation of the starved heart model. Deprived of magnesium (usually as the result of stress), your heart cannot produce enough energy; without energy, your heart, arteries, and veins quickly begin to deteriorate, leading to heart cell death. In turn, heart cell death leads to calcification, and calcification to the inflammation that Fuster and Libby observed. Moreover, research has shown that magnesium deficiency independently plays a role in many critical heart conditions, ranging from arrhythmia to heart attack. Both directly and indirectly, magnesium starvation is at the very core of heart disease.

Accordingly, by taking steps to avoid or rectify magnesium deficiency, you can help stop heart disease before it even starts. Research shows that by maintaining optimal levels of magnesium, you can protect against heart disease, preventing or decreasing your risk of heart attacks, stroke, and high blood pressure (hypertension). Simply put, magnesium is the most essential nutrient for promoting and maintaining proper heart function.

A Closer Look at the Starved Heart Model

As this brief overview indicates, the starved heart model asserts that heart disease is the end result of a degenerative process initiated by lack of magnesium. In order to properly understand this process—and how magnesium deficiency is integral to every part of it—this section breaks down the starved heart model into simple, easy-to-understand steps. For a quick reference guide, please see the chart on page 96.

Stress

What causes magnesium deficiency in the first place? As detailed in Chapter 2, the primary source of magnesium deficiency is stress. Stress evolved as a way for primitive humans to cope with perceived threats. When confronted with an immediate danger (say, a hungry lion looking for its next meal), the bodies of your ancient ancestors released stress hormones—including epinephrine (adrenaline), cortisol, and aldosterone—that allowed them to either fight their foe or run away from it. This "fight-or-flight" response is an evolutionary gift, a survival mechanism that has historically allowed humans to thrive and avoid extinction.

These days, most of us don't face grave bodily harm. Instead, stressors are more likely to be psychological or emotional in nature, though various physical conditions (exposure to toxic chemicals or metals, nutrient-deprived food) can also put your body under strain. Worse still, stress tends to be long term, or chronic—you can kill or run away from a lion, but it's much harder to cope with a bad relationship or a high-pressure job.

Whatever the source of the stress, your bodily response remains the same as that of your ancient ancestors: you release stress hormones. The longer you endure stress, the more stress hormones your body produces. And the more stress hormones your body produces, the more magnesium your body uses up. This is because magnesium regulates and controls hormone production; when your body is flooded with cortisol and other stress hormones, magnesium is quickly expended in an effort to bring levels down to normal. Without magnesium, your stress hormone levels will remain elevated for an extended period of time. The result of chronic stress, therefore, is chronic magnesium deficiency.

Magnesium Deficiency

Magnesium deficiency is a serious condition that can have many implications for your health—and your heart health in particular. As explained in Chapter 2, magnesium performs many roles in your body. It acts as a cofactor for various vitamins, minerals, enzymes, and other compounds, activating them and allowing them to carry out more than a thousand different chemical reactions that are necessary for your body to function properly. Without magnesium, your body simply cannot carry out the vital processes that allow you to conduct your daily activities.

Magnesium deficiency is particularly hard on your heart. Here are some of the heart-related functions that magnesium performs under optimal circumstances:

- Aids in detoxification and protects against the accumulation of environmental toxins and free radicals in the cells and tissues, thus protecting the arteries from potential sources of damage.

- Assists in the process by which DNA is copied and repaired, thus aiding in proper cell division, cell maintenance, and cell repair, allowing for proper generation and maintenance of heart muscle cells.

- Dilates blood vessels, making it easier for the heart to pump blood and more effectively transmit nutrients and oxygen to the body's cells, tissues, and organs.

- Enhances immune function and helps protect against infection, which has been linked to an increased risk of heart disease.

- Helps regulate blood pressure and protects against spasms in the artery walls.

- Prevents the formation of dangerous blood clots that can obstruct the arteries.

More important, magnesium plays an essential role in both regulating the calcium in your body and producing the energy (Mg-ATP) your body needs to function. Without magnesium, these two vital processes cannot be maintained; the results of this failure can potentially be disastrous for your heart and cardiovascular system.

Electrolyte Imbalance. One of magnesium's most critical jobs is to regulate calcium. As discussed in Chapter 3, magnesium and calcium are two electrolytes (charged molecules) that are forever engaged in a dynamic balancing act within your cells. Both electrolytes are important for good health, yet they act as biological antagonists to each other, the presence of one offsetting the presence of the other. When magnesium and calcium are not in balance —as in a state of magnesium deficiency—a wide range of health problems and chronic illnesses unfold, most notably heart disease.

At the cellular level, magnesium acts as a sort of gatekeeper, making sure that excess calcium doesn't enter the interior of your cells. Magnesium acts as a natural calcium blocker; if magnesium isn't available, calcium floods your cells, creating an electrolyte imbalance that can induce several serious heart conditions, including arrhythmia, angina, premature ventricular contraction, and hypertension.

Outside the cells, magnesium also helps regulate calcium by activating three hormones that control the level and location of calcium inside your body. Without an adequate supply of magnesium, these hormones are unable to properly perform their tasks. The result is that calcium accumulates and migrates to areas of the body where it does not belong—including your arteries, where deposits build up and contribute to atherosclerosis.

Worse still, excess calcium can activate your sympathetic nervous system (SNS). The SNS is the body system that controls your automatic, unconscious functioning; it is responsible for initiating both the "fight-or-flight" response and the inflammatory process. Without magnesium to check its presence, calcium overstimulates your SNS, triggering the inflammatory cascade that Peter Libby described in the chronic inflammation model. By stimulating the SNS, excess calcium also increases your already-high levels of stress hormones, creating a vicious circle: stress leads to magnesium deficiency, which leads to electrolyte imbalance balance, which leads to more stress!

Ideally, your body would attain a balanced ratio of magnesium to calcium, as discussed in Chapter 2. Unfortunately, even with an adequate intake of magnesium, it is very difficult to keep magnesium and calcium in equilibrium. Human biochemistry has evolved in such a way that the body is predisposed to hold onto as much calcium as possible, while simultaneously letting go of magnesium. Moreover, doctors frequently recommend that patients get more calcium in order to ward off osteoporosis and other ailments; as a result, the average American today tends to receive about ten times as much calcium as magnesium through diet and supplements. Factoring in magnesium depletion as a result of stress, it is hardly surprising that the vast majority of Americans suffer from heart-hurting electrolyte imbalances.

Decline in Energy Production. Another serious consequence of magnesium deficiency is a decline in energy production. Without magnesium, your heart also cannot make the energy it needs to work properly. Adenosine triphosphate (ATP) is the basic energy currency of your body's cells; it enables most, if not all, of your body's fundamental metabolic processes. But, as explained in Chapter 2, in order to carry out these vital processes, ATP first must be activated by magnesium. Under normal circumstances, free magnesium ions bind to an ATP molecule, forming a new compound called Mg-ATP that has a different shape and electrical charge, making it easier for the energy within to be accessed and used by your cells.

All of your heart's 100 trillion cells need Mg-ATP in order to function, and your heart muscle cells are no exception. In fact, because your heart works harder than any other organ in the body, it needs the most Mg-ATP—and therefore the most magnesium. When your heart is deprived of magnesium, it cannot produce enough Mg-ATP. Without Mg-ATP, your heart muscle cells lack the energy to contract, and their ability to pump blood through your system is impaired.

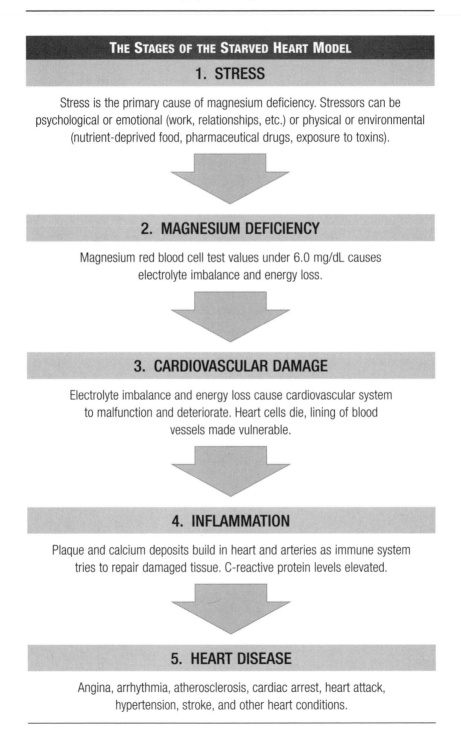

THE STAGES OF THE STARVED HEART MODEL

1. STRESS

Stress is the primary cause of magnesium deficiency. Stressors can be psychological or emotional (work, relationships, etc.) or physical or environmental (nutrient-deprived food, pharmaceutical drugs, exposure to toxins).

2. MAGNESIUM DEFICIENCY

Magnesium red blood cell test values under 6.0 mg/dL causes electrolyte imbalance and energy loss.

3. CARDIOVASCULAR DAMAGE

Electrolyte imbalance and energy loss cause cardiovascular system to malfunction and deteriorate. Heart cells die, lining of blood vessels made vulnerable.

4. INFLAMMATION

Plaque and calcium deposits build in heart and arteries as immune system tries to repair damaged tissue. C-reactive protein levels elevated.

5. HEART DISEASE

Angina, arrhythmia, atherosclerosis, cardiac arrest, heart attack, hypertension, stroke, and other heart conditions.

Heart Cell Death and Artery Damage

As a result of both electrolyte imbalance and energy loss, your cardiovascular system begins to deteriorate. If your heart goes without Mg-ATP for prolonged periods of time, your heart cells begin to starve and die. This heart cell death (cardiac necrosis) can be one of the most devastating consequences of magnesium deficiency. But that's not all. Research has shown that magnesium deficiency doesn't just affect your heart cells; it also contributes to endothelial dysfunction, a condition in which the lining of your blood vessels is either injured or impaired. Without sufficient magnesium to regulate the levels of other electrolytes, calcium builds up in the interior of your cells, undermining their structural soundness and causing damage. In other words, magnesium deficiency compromises the integrity of your cardiovascular system from the cellular level on up.

Inflammation

With your heart cells dying and the lining of your blood vessels potentially damaged, inflammation sets in—if it hasn't already in reaction to the electrolyte imbalance. As explained earlier, inflammation is essentially an immune response, designed to heal injured tissue. When your body senses a dead (necrotic) area or a wound in your arteries or heart, it sends remedial agents to repair and close the breach: blood cells, cholesterol, and different minerals, including calcium. These agents accumulate in the wall of the heart or arteries, forming the composite substance known as vulnerable plaque. Sometimes, the whole area contracts and scars, leaving tough, fibrous tissue where healthy tissue once existed. And, without sufficient magnesium to regulate the levels of free calcium in your blood, deposits of this mineral also build up in your arteries and heart, leading to new obstructions and hardened tissue.

Heart Disease

As Fuster and Libby have shown, the end result of the inflammatory process is atherosclerosis and thrombosis, which in turn lead to the development of other heart diseases, including angina, heart attack, and stroke. Atherosclerosis arises when plaque builds up in your arteries, compromising the arteries' ability to pump blood throughout your body, thus contributing to hypertension and angina. Thrombosis occurs when clots form in your blood vessels, preventing or limiting blood flow and potentially causing heart attack or stroke.

The important thing to remember here is that the entire sequence of events—from electrolyte imbalance to energy loss to cell death to inflammation to heart disease—is affected by magnesium deficiency. Furthermore, magnesium deficiency plays a role in every stage in the development of heart ailments, contributing to and often compounding the disease conditions.

The Evolution of the Starved Heart Model

The starved heart model is a relatively new theory developed by independent researcher Morley Robbins. The name of the theory comes from the Harvard scientist Joanne Ingwall, who in 1993 was the first to formally propose the idea that the heart is a metabolic powerhouse that depends on ATP for energy. Over the last two decades, Ingwall has devoted her research to showing that when deprived of this energy, the heart starves, a condition that leads to cell death and, eventually, disease.

But the theoretical origins of the starved heart model of heart disease go much further back, to Karl Ludwig Alfred Fiedler, an Austrian physician who was active in the early 1900s. Building on the work of Rudolf Virchow fifty years earlier, Fiedler hypothesized that heart disease follows three distinct phases: cardiac necrosis (heart cell death), inflammation, and then calcification. This idea was more thoroughly developed in the 1950s by Hans Selye, who is primarily known today as the first researcher to demonstrate the existence and effects of biological stress.

Selye's work on stress extended to its effects on heart health. In 1958, Selye published his groundbreaking treatise *The Chemical Prevention of Cardiac Necrosis.* In it, he established that the true cause of heart disease was stress, which led to heart cell death, inflammation, and fibrosis/calcification. Only after a critical mass of cells die, Selye pointed out, does the process of heart disease truly begin.

In effect, Selye was saying that heart disease follows inflammation and atherosclerosis. For the first time in history, Selye was offering a viable model of heart disease that truly got at the cause of heart disease, not its effects. Perhaps even more significantly, Selye's findings indicated that the effects of stress on your heart could be limited and even prevented by the use of magnesium supplements.

This idea was expanded upon by the pioneering researcher Mildred S. Seelig, a former president of the American College of Nutrition who spent more than fifty years researching the roles played by magnesium deficiencies in the development of disease. More than any other doctor or scientist, Seelig is responsible for drawing attention to magnesium as an important ingredient for good health, and for pointing out the connection between magnesium deficiency and cardiovascular disease. Seelig's research also clearly established the direct link between stress and magnesium loss. Her findings demonstrated that ongoing exposure to stress and the resultant loss of magnesium leads to a vicious cycle that can significantly and rapidly deplete magnesium stores in the muscular tissue of the heart (myocardium), causing damage and allowing a dangerous influx of calcium into the interior of the heart cells, where it does not belong. Refining Selye's work, Seelig showed that the end result of this magnesium depletion is heart cell death.

Increasingly, other scientists and doctors have begun to validate Seelig's work. Burton and Bella Altura have done extensive work on the tendency of magnesium deficiency to cause vasospasms, or spasms in the blood vessels—a condition that has vast implications for a variety of heart conditions, including angina, hypertension, and heart attack. Significant research has also been conducted by cardiologist William Weglicki, former president of the North American division of the International Society for Heart Research. Since the 1990s, Weglicki has explored the ways by which heart disease is affected or caused by magnesium deficiency. Specifically, Weglicki has established the important link between low magnesium and inflammation, the precursor to many heart conditions and other health problems. Weglicki highlighted magnesium's role as a regulator of calcium, and showed that an imbalanced ratio of calcium to magnesium triggers the inflammatory response that can be so damaging to the heart.

Together, these scientists have helped to create a firm foundation for the starved heart model, convincingly demonstrating that magnesium deficiency is a prime culprit in the electrolyte imbalance, energy depletion, cell death, and inflammation that leads to heart disease.

Evidence for the Starved Heart Model

In response to the work of Seelig, Weglicki, and the Alturas, the medical community has increasingly begun to give credence to the idea that magnesium deficiency is an important factor in the development of cardiovascular disease. Over the last two decades, compelling new research has begun to accumulate in support of the starved heart model. This section offers just a few examples from this growing body of work:

- A 1992 study published in the *American Heart Journal* reported that sudden death is common in areas where community water supplies are magnesium deficient; that people who die of sudden death caused by heart disease are more likely to have low magnesium levels in their heart cells; that cardiac arrhythmias and coronary artery spasms can be caused by magnesium deficiency; and that magnesium administered intravenously reduces the risk of arrhythmia and death immediately after heart attack.

- A 1992 study overseen by the Alturas and published in the journal *Magnesium and Trace Elements* found that blood levels of magnesium help determine the integrity and responsiveness of human blood vessels, and accordingly that low blood levels of magnesium result in a higher risk of ischemic heart disease, heart disease, atherosclerosis, and arterial spasms.

- A 1994 study published in the journal *Magnesium Research* reported that magnesium supplementation led to "an impressive decrease" in the frequency of angina attacks in patients who already suffered from this disease.

- A 1995 study published in the *Journal of the American College of Nutrition* reported that low magnesium levels are "significantly and inversely associated with coronary heart and vascular disease deaths and hospitalizations," meaning that the risks for coronary heart disease and atherosclerosis increase as magnesium levels decrease.

- A comprehensive review published in 2012 by the *American Journal for Clinical Nutrition* examined previous studies involving more than 241,000 participants and found a "statistically significant inverse association between magnesium intake and risk of stroke." In other words, the less magnesium in your body, the greater your risk for stroke.

- Also in 2012, Weglicki published an overview of animal and human studies in the journal *Circulation,* establishing a causative link between low magnesium levels and inflammation and showing that levels of C-reactive protein (the primary chemical marker used to evaluate inflammation) were consistently higher in adults who consumed less than half the DRI (Dietary Reference Intakes) of magnesium. Weglicki also asserted that low magnesium levels were associated with higher risk for arrhythmia, angina, and hypertension; and that low magnesium levels were frequently found in subjects suffering from obesity and/or metabolic syndrome (see Chapter 5).

- In 2013, a study published in the journal *Hypertension,* researchers found that each one-unit (1.0 mg/dL) increase in the blood concentration of magnesium resulted in a 21 percent decrease in the risk of developing hypertension.

- In another 2013 study published in the *American Journal of Clinical Nutrition,* researchers periodically measured the magnesium levels of 7,664 test subjects with no prior history of heart disease over ten years. The researchers found that those with the lowest magnesium levels had a 60 percent greater risk of developing ischemic (oxygen-deprived) heart disease, and 70 percent greater likelihood of dying from it.

One of the most important studies to recognize magnesium's relationship to heart disease is the Atherosclerosis Risk in Communities (ARIC) study, begun in 1987, with results and analyses published on a consistent basis in the *American Heart Journal* and elsewhere. This ongoing study follows over 14,000 test subjects between the ages of forty-five to sixty-four in order to assess dietary and other risk factors for different forms of heart disease. Analysis from this study shows magnesium deficiency is a significant risk factor for many serious heart conditions, including atherosclerosis, cardiac arrest, coronary heart disease, and coronary thrombosis—and is also an independent risk factor for several conditions that contribute to heart disease, including type 2 diabetes and metabolic syndrome.

Most recently, researchers from Harvard University's School of Public Health published a review of sixteen earlier studies with a combined subject pool of over 300,000 people. The purpose of the review was to determine what role, if any, dietary magnesium plays in reducing the risk of cardiovascular disease. After analyzing the sixteen studies, the researchers found that the data overwhelmingly pointed to a significant link between magnesium and heart disease. In review, they found that increased dietary intake of magnesium reduces the overall risk of cardiovascular disease by as much as 30 percent, and reduces the risk of heart disease due specifically to oxygen loss by 22 percent.

The Harvard researchers ended their review with a call for more clinical trials to determine whether magnesium could be effective in treating and preventing cardiovascular disease. This initiative should be supported—any work that examines magnesium's benefits for heart disease can raise awareness of this mineral and thus potentially save lives. As the studies continue to pour in, the evidence seems clear and unambiguous: Because magnesium deficiency is such an important determinant of heart disease, magnesium supplementation can play a definite and primary role in heart disease prevention.

CONCLUSION

Having read this chapter, you now have a better understanding of how heart disease develops—and what you can do about it. An emerging model that attempts to explain the origins of heart disease is the starved heart model, which asserts that the heart that is starved for magnesium is a heart that cannot produce enough energy, clearing the pathways to inflammation and eventually cardiovascular disease. The underlying cause—the missing link that may explain why so many Americans today die of heart disease—is magnesium deficiency.

Despite the preponderance of evidence currently available, most doctors are only recently beginning to pay attention to the role of magnesium in heart disease. When the dust finally settles regarding the research on hypertension, cardiomyopathy, congestive heart failure, arrhythmia, premature ventricular contractions, heart attacks, and cardiac arrest, one thing will be clear—that magnesium deficiency is involved in every one of these cardiovascular conditions.

It may take years for the medical community to get wise to the importance of magnesium for your heart. But you need not wait in order to reap the advantages of this powerful mineral. In the chapter that follows, you'll learn of magnesium's benefits for other diseases, including type 2 diabetes, chronic fatigue, fibromyalgia, and insomnia. Then, Chapter 6 will provide you with a practical guide to optimizing your magnesium levels.

If magnesium deficiency is the root cause of heart disease, the solution is simple. Address the problem at the source! By making sure that you never lack for magnesium, you can significantly reduce your risk of developing heart disease. Protect yourself—the power is in your hands!

5

Magnesium's Other Health Benefits

Although this book focuses on magnesium's capacity to both prevent and help reverse heart disease, it is important to note that magnesium has advantages for many other areas of your health. In fact, an understanding of this miraculous nutrient will change the way you view—and treat—many of our nation's most common conditions and diseases. Magnesium deficiency underlies countless pressing health issues; accordingly, magnesium supplementation can do much to either prevent or remedy them. In addition, supplementation can improve conditions for which magnesium deficiency is not a direct factor. The benefits of magnesium are powerful and wide-ranging.

This chapter explores the role played by magnesium in some of the most widespread health epidemics that face Americans today, including obesity, diabetes, depression, gastrointestinal disorders, and sleep issues. While magnesium cannot solve all your problems, it can certainly be a valuable addition to your daily regimen, particularly if you suffer from any of the conditions discussed below.

OBESITY, DIABETES, AND METABOLIC SYNDROME

One hundred years ago, obesity, type 2 diabetes, and metabolic syndrome were all virtually nonexistent in our nation. Now, however, these conditions have become more common with each passing year. Not only are obesity, diabetes, and metabolic syndrome dangerous on their own, but each of these conditions also raises its sufferer's risk for developing heart disease and other serious conditions, including cancer.

All three of these conditions are generally known as lifestyle diseases, meaning that their development is closely linked to eating habits and other behavioral choices, including exercise, or the lack thereof. It is interesting to note that the increased incidence of these conditions parallels the steady decline of magnesium in our nation's soil and food supply, along with the progressive development of other magnesium-robbing factors, as discussed in Chapter 2.

One point that is important to emphasize about these three conditions is that they are all interrelated. Obesity and metabolic syndrome are risk factors for diabetes, and at the same time, the insulin resistance that characterizes type 2 diabetes is also independently associated with metabolic syndrome and obesity. This is no coincidence: All three conditions are in actuality manifestations of the same underlying factors. While magnesium deficiency is not the sole cause of these conditions, it certainly plays a major role in their development and progression. Let's take a closer look at each condition so that you can better understand why this is so.

Obesity

The statistics on obesity are staggering. According to the Centers for Disease Control and Prevention (CDC), approximately 17 percent of all American children between the ages of two and nineteen are currently obese. That's 12.5 million children—triple the number recorded in 1980. In adults, the problem is even worse. According to the CDC, 35.7 percent of all men and women in the United States are obese. Two decades ago, not a single state in the nation had an obesity rate higher than 15 percent. Today, every state does, with twelve states having obesity rates of 30 percent or more. All told, Americans are overweight by a collective 4.5 billion pounds. And this trend shows no signs of reversing itself—an additional 30 percent of Americans are classified as overweight.

New research indicates that weight gain is not simply a matter of consuming more calories than you burn. In fact, there are a number of more important factors implicated in unhealthy weight gain. It's no coincidence that studies have consistently shown that magnesium levels are lower in people who are overweight or obese than they are in people of normal weight. Among the factors scientists have consistently linked to obesity are chronic stress, insulin resistance, and inflammation—three conditions that are also heavily associated with magnesium deficiency.

Stress can contribute to obesity in a number of ways, most notably by interfering with your metabolism. During an acute or momentary episode of stress, your body releases a hormone called cortisol. In order to provide your body with the fuel it needs to power its "fight-or-flight" response, cortisol stimulates the production of certain hormones that turn your existing food stores into energy, including insulin, which processes glucose (sugar). In the short term, thus, cortisol might be seen as preventing weight gain, since it essentially speeds up your metabolism.

In the long term, however, stress can have the opposite effect. When you are exposed to chronic stress, your body is flooded with insulin; over time, however, your body becomes used to its presence and loses the ability to respond to it, developing a condition called insulin resistance. The result is that you continue to eat, but fail to properly process the contents of your food. Your metabolism slows, you burn through fewer calories, and you gain weight.

As discussed in Chapter 2, magnesium can help you regulate stress. By increasing your magnesium intake, you can buffer the effects of cortisol, and thus help avoid weight gain. If you don't increase your magnesium intake during stressful periods, cortisol will run rampant, advancing insulin resistance. To make matters worse, as previously noted, chronic stress causes magnesium deficiency, which in itself contributes to insulin resistance, because magnesium helps to control the production and regulate the activity of insulin.

Magnesium deficiency also underlies another critical factor in weight gain: inflammation. A recent study showed that obesity is often characterized by the presence of chronic low-grade inflammation, and, in turn, that inflammation seems to be either caused or exacerbated by low magnesium levels. Evidence suggests that chronic inflammation can affect the proper functioning of the hypothalamus, the part of your brain that controls your hunger response. When the hypothalamus is inflamed, you lose your ability to regulate cravings and normal eating habits; the result is weight gain.

Help is available. By maintaining adequate levels of magnesium, you will improve your overall capacity to control the effects of stress and inflammation on your metabolism. Research also shows that increasing magnesium levels through diet or oral magnesium supplements directly reduces insulin resistance, even in people with normal levels of magnesium.

Of course, magnesium by itself is not a magic bullet for weight loss. If you are overweight, simply increasing your magnesium intake alone will not be enough to shed your unwanted pounds. You will also need to engage in moderate daily physical activity— a thirty-minute walk each day will suffice for most people. Avoid overeating, and instead, eat healthily: Cut out sugar, sodas, and all simple white carbohydrate foods and minimize your intake of complex carbohydrates, as high-carbohydrate intake depletes magnesium. Manage your stress levels, and get adequate amounts of sleep each night. But if you've already been doing all of these things with little to show for it, now you know why. Increase your magnesium intake and see results!

Type 2 Diabetes

Type 2 diabetes is a chronic condition in which your body has difficulty making or using insulin, a hormone that, as previously discussed, helps your body metabolize or make use of glucose (sugar), our main source of fuel. Unlike type 1 diabetes, in which the pancreas is damaged by the immune system, in type 2 diabetes the pancreas is intact, but either the amount of insulin produced is insufficient or the body fails to respond to its effects, developing a condition called insulin resistance. If left untreated, type 2 diabetes can be life-threatening.

The incidence of type 2 diabetes in the United States rises with each passing year. Even more troubling is the fact that in the last two decades, there has been a dramatic spike in the number of children and adolescents who have developed type 2 diabetes—an increase that parallels and corresponds to the growth in obesity rates for both groups. While doctors once thought type 2 diabetes only developed in older people, calling it "adult-onset diabetes," as more children and adolescents are diagnosed, it is now quite clear that this disease can occur at any age.

The rise of type 2 diabetes parallels the rise in magnesium deficiency. This is no coincidence; in fact, according to Dr. Jerry Nadler of the Eastern Virginia Medical School, diabetes is "a magnesium deficiency state."

Research has established that magnesium levels of diabetic patients tend to be much lower than normal, with at least 90 percent of all diabetes patients classified as magnesium deficient. Aside from diet, one possible explanation for this deficiency is that diabetics excrete more magnesium through their urine than nondiabetics do. This means that their need for magnesium in diabetics is even greater than it is for most other people because they lose magnesium at a faster rate than others do. Research has indicated that lack of magnesium also underlies the development of other problems suffered as a consequence of diabetes, including retinopathy (damage to the blood vessels of the eye), altered glucose levels, high blood pressure, and abnormal platelet function.

A study conducted by the American Diabetes Association (ADA) supported the use of magnesium supplements to improve the symptoms of type 2 diabetes. Specifically, the study proved that magnesium supplementation improves insulin sensitivity and blood glucose control in diabetic subjects with low magnesium levels. As a result of the study, the ADA published a consensus statement recommending that patients with diabetes who have low levels of magnesium take magnesium supplements.

These findings were supported by two large-scale studies conducted by researchers at the Harvard Medical School and School of Public Health. In the first study, approximately 85,000 female and 42,000 male test subjects were followed for eighteen and twelve years, respectively. During that time, about 5,400 people developed diabetes. Even after taking into account other diabetes risk factors (age, weight, physical activity, smoking, and family history), the study found that those study participants who consumed the most magnesium-rich foods had significantly lower risk for diabetes when compared with those who consumed less magnesium-rich food. The level of risk remained the same even after researchers adjusted for other dietary factors such as the fat and fiber content of foods and their glycemic load. The second study, involving nearly 40,000 women age forty-five or older, showed similar results.

The evidence is clear: Increase your intake of magnesium, and reduce your risk of developing type 2 diabetes. If you already have type 2 diabetes, check with your doctor first before beginning a supplementation program; because kidney function is impaired in some diabetics, you may have difficulty excreting excess amounts of magnesium.

Metabolic Syndrome

Also known as syndrome X or insulin resistance syndrome, metabolic syndrome refers to a combination of health disorders that collectively increase the risk for not only obesity and diabetes, but also heart attack, stroke, and other types of heart disease. Metabolic syndrome is characterized by four conditions:

- Hyperlipidemia—high levels of triglycerides or fats in your blood

- Hypertension—high blood pressure

- Hyperglycemia—high blood sugar

- Imbalances or irregularities in the hypothalamic, pituitary, and adrenal glands

Typically, you need to have at least three of these conditions in order to be diagnosed with metabolic syndrome; however, any one of these conditions increases your risk of developing heart disease, and the more of them you have, the greater your overall risk is.

According to the American Diabetes Association, over 34 percent of Americans suffer from metabolic syndrome, many of them unknowingly. And this rate is likely to rise, as metabolic syndrome is a risk factor for obesity and type 2 diabetes—both conditions that have seen statistical increases as well. While metabolic syndrome was previously believed to predominantly affect men, in recent years, rates of incidence have already increased for women, children, and adolescents. Older people have a higher risk for metabolic syndrome, as do Asians and Latinos.

Given the role that magnesium deficiency plays in both obesity and diabetes, it's not surprising that lack of magnesium also significantly increases the risk for metabolic syndrome. When magnesium levels are low, the proper balance between magnesium and calcium is thrown out of kilter. As you learned in Chapter 4, magnesium is the gatekeeper that regulates the level of calcium inside your cells; when your body doesn't receive enough magnesium, excess calcium builds up inside your body's 100 trillion cells. And, as Drs. Lawrence M. Resnick and Mildred S. Seelig have shown, this excess calcium leads to metabolic syndrome.

A fifteen-year study of over 4,600 people between the ages of eighteen and thirty found that people who ate the highest amounts of magnesium-rich foods reduced their risk of developing metabolic syndrome by as much as 31 percent. No doubt the risk would be further reduced by adding magnesium supplementation to a diet rich in magnesium foods.

The relationship between magnesium deficiency and metabolic syndrome has been confirmed in other studies as well. In one, 192 men and women with metabolic syndrome were compared to a control group of 384 healthy adults to determine the relationship between magnesium deficiency and metabolic syndrome. Tellingly, however, researchers found that over 65 percent of test subjects with metabolic syndrome suffered from

Magnesium Protects Our Nation's Children

The incidence of obesity is increasing at an alarming rate among our children, and as a result, the incidences of type 2 diabetes and metabolic syndrome are increasing as well. Although research had previously established that magnesium deficiency is a characteristic of nearly all adults who suffer from insulin resistance and impaired glucose regulation, it wasn't until 2005 that researchers at the University of Virginia confirmed that the same phenomenon existed in children.

In a study to determine the relationship between magnesium deficiency and insulin resistance in obese children, researchers found that 55 percent of obese children between the ages of eight and seventeen did not get enough magnesium from the foods they ate, compared with 27 percent of lean children. Not only did the obese children not eat enough foods rich in magnesium, but they also exhibited problems in the way their bodies made use of the dietary magnesium they did get. Researchers discovered that the obese children actually derived 14.4 percent less magnesium from the foods they ate than lean children did, even though obese and lean children ate about the same number of calories per day. As a result, the obese children had much lower magnesium levels in their blood than the lean children. Most important, the obese children were found to also suffer from insulin resistance in direct proportion to how to the severity of their magnesium deficiency.

The findings of this study cannot be overemphasized, because they provide us with a simple and easy solution for preventing three of our nation's most serious disease epidemics. By ensuring that our children get all the magnesium they need up to and throughout adulthood, we could conceivably reverse the trend of childhood obesity and wipe out both type 2 diabetes and metabolic syndrome within a generation.

magnesium deficiency, compared with less than 5 percent of the control group. The study concluded that not only was there a strong overall correlation between magnesium deficiency and metabolic syndrome, but that magnesium deficiency was separately indicated in two of the preconditions of metabolic syndrome, hyperlipidemia and high blood pressure, and could also be considered an independent risk factor for type 2 diabetes.

The discussion of obesity, diabetes, and metabolic syndrome was begun by pointing out how pervasive these conditions are in modern-day society, and how each of them significantly increases your risk of heart disease. Now that you have read this far, you know how magnesium can prevent or help to reverse each of these conditions. By increasing awareness of magnesium's importance, before long, we can return to a time when all three of these conditions are virtually nonexistent.

OTHER COMMON HEALTH CONDITIONS THAT BENEFIT FROM MAGNESIUM

Besides obesity, type 2 diabetes, and metabolic syndrome, there are a lot of other health conditions to which magnesium deficiency can contribute. These conditions can also benefit greatly from magnesium supplementation. This section will examine some of the most common health issues in which magnesium plays a role.

Depression

Depression is a psychological condition that can have serious consequences if left untreated. It is characterized by feelings of sadness and disinterest in one's daily life. Severe cases of depression can lead to a withdrawal from friends and family, prolonged fatigue, feelings of futility, irrational outbursts of anger, and even suicide. Chronic depression can also trigger a wide variety of physical symptoms, including loss of appetite, compulsive overeating, gastrointestinal problems, sleeping problems, back pain, and headaches. If you or your loved ones suffer from prolonged bouts of depression, seek prompt medical attention and the help of a skilled therapist or counselor trained to deal with such issues.

While magnesium is certainly not a complete solution for depression, research does indicate that it can be very helpful for easing the symptoms, potentially resolving them completely and reducing the risk of their recurrence. In fact, because of the mental health benefits magnesium can provide, Dr. Emily Deans, a practicing psychiatrist, referred to it as "the original chill pill" in an article published online by *Psychology Today*. As she wrote, "When you start to untangle the effects of magnesium in the nervous system, you touch upon nearly every single biological mechanism for depression."

Magnesium helps to protect against depression in a number of ways. First, when present in the body in optimal amounts, it regulates the activity of both calcium and glutamate, which are found in the synapses between the cells of the nervous system, or neurons. Among other functions, calcium and glutamate serve to activate a part of the neuron called the N-methyl D-aspartate (NMDA) receptor, which plays a role in both memory function and the ability of the synapses to adapt in response to nerve impulses. When levels of magnesium are low, calcium and glutamate build up, triggering the NMDA receptor too frequently. This excess activity in the NMDA receptor is correlated with higher rates of both anxiety and depression. In addition, this activity can also lead to neuron damage or death. As George and Karen Eby write, "Without magnesium, the neuron operates much like an automobile without brakes, blasting calcium through the synapses, causing great harm to the brain, with severe disruption of thinking, mood and behavior." Sufficient levels of magnesium prevent this cascade of events from happening by regulating the calcium and glutamate that cause the initial damage.

The second way by which magnesium protects against anxiety and depression has to do with its ability to buffer the effects of stress. As this chapter shows, long-term exposure to stress can result in sleep disorders and chronic inflammation, both of which are independent risk factors for anxiety and depression. In addition, the brain's memory center, the hippocampus, is particularly sensitive to the stress hormone cortisol. When exposed to excess levels of that stress hormone, the hippocampus can become damaged or even atrophy—waste away. Recent studies have shown that this smaller or partially impaired hippocampus is highly correlated with major depressive disorder.

How can magnesium help? As explained previously, magnesium helps regulate cortisol, effectively buffering the effects of stress and limiting the toll it takes on your body and brain. In a research paper, the Ebys examined multiple case histories of patients who suffered from major depression, and found that all of the patients experienced rapid recovery in less than seven days after using 125 to 300 milligrams of magnesium with each meal and at bedtime. They also found that magnesium supplementation improved related mental illnesses, including traumatic brain injury, headache, suicidal ideation, anxiety, irritability, insomnia, postpartum depression, cocaine, alcohol and tobacco abuse, hypersensitivity to calcium, short-term memory loss, and IQ loss. Clearly, magnesium has enormous significance for the treatment of psychological disorders.

Asthma

Asthma is a chronic lung disease in which the airways are inflamed and narrowed, making it difficult to breathe and causing coughing, wheezing, and shortness of breath. The incidence of asthma has increased over the last few decades, particularly among the young. Researchers estimate that up to 15 percent of all children in the United States now suffer from asthma. This statistic is sad, but not surprising, as the rise of asthma corresponds to the decline of magnesium in our food supply.

Magnesium can be useful in preventing and treating asthma. Many studies have linked magnesium deficiency to lung dysfunction, and magnesium sufficiency to improved lung function. Asthma is triggered when levels of histamines and stress hormones become elevated, causing muscle spasms and inflammation and thus narrowing the airways. Magnesium helps control the release of histamines and stress hormones, keeps your muscles relaxed, and more generally prevents unhealthy inflammation. Because of these properties, magnesium can actually stop an asthma attack as it occurs. Conversely, lack of magnesium can leave your body more vulnerable to an attack.

In a study of over 2,500 children between the ages of eleven and ninteen, researchers found that low magnesium levels were correlated with a reduction in overall lung function, decreasing lung capacity and the flow of air through the respiratory system. Another study examined the effects of magnesium supplementation on patients who suffered with mild to moderate asthma. After six months, patients who had taken 170 milligrams of magnesium citrate twice a day showed improvement in the frequency and severity of asthma attacks, performed better on pulmonary function tests, and generally were seen to have higher quality of life.

Clearly, magnesium has a number of benefits for asthmatics. An adequate supply of magnesium in the body helps to keep the muscles of the respiratory system relaxed and dilated, facilitating breathing. Magnesium has also been shown to reduce histamine and inflammation levels in the lungs and overall respiratory system, thus helping to prevent the recurrence of asthma attacks. These beneficial properties of magnesium explain why magnesium is administered intravenously in hospitals to treat the symptoms of life-threatening, drug-resistant asthma attacks. Unfortunately, many of the medications typically prescribed to treat asthma often worsen the condition. One of the most notorious side effects of these drugs, which are used to open respiratory pathways and reduce inflammation in the lungs and nasal passages, is the depletion of magnesium in the body. While quick-relief asthma drugs can certainly be valuable in cases of severe asthma attacks, patients should be weaned off of long-term medications, while simultaneously increasing their magnesium intake in order to improve overall lung function.

Chronic Fatigue and
Chronic Fatigue Syndrome (CFS)

Chronic fatigue, or chronic fatigue syndrome (CFS), is one of the most common health complaints. It is characterized not only by debilitating fatigue, but also a range of other symptoms, including headaches, swollen glands, periodic fevers and chills, muscle and joint aches and pains, muscle weakness, sore throat, and numbness and tingling of the extremities. The primary symptom is a state of severe fatigue that makes doing even the simplest of tasks an exhausting proposition. Considering that nearly everyone in the United States today is deficient in magnesium, the preponderance of chronic fatigue syndrome is hardly surprising. Why? Because, as explained in Chapter 4, magnesium is by far the most important nutrient needed by your body to produce energy at the cellular level.

Briefly, let's review how your body produces energy. Inside each of your body's 100 trillion cells are tiny energy factories called mitochondria. The job of the mitochondria is to create energy by breaking down glucose and other compounds to release a useable cellular fuel called adenosine triphosphate, or ATP. ATP acts as an instant source of energy within the cell, powering all of your body's energy-consuming functions. Without magnesium, the mitochondria can't do their job. No magnesium means impaired mitochondria function. Impaired mitochondria means no ATP. No ATP means no energy. It's that simple.

Not only is magnesium essential for the production of ATP—it's also important for maintaining the stability and functionality of ATP once it's produced. As discussed earlier, the substance that we commonly refer to as ATP is actually the compound magnesium-ATP, or Mg-ATP. Without its magnesium attachment, ATP quickly begins to break down into less stable, and therefore less usable, compounds.

In other words, without enough magnesium to draw upon, you cannot get the energy you need to conduct your daily life, and will necessarily suffer from fatigue. When you suffer from fatigue, your body's need for magnesium becomes even greater. Chronic fatigue and magnesium deficiency thus form a vicious cycle.

Although there are many causes of CFS, there is no doubt that magnesium deficiency is a major factor. In 1991, two studies on the relationship between magnesium deficiency and CFS were published in the prestigious medical journal *Lancet*. In both studies, test subjects with CFS were found to have low magnesium levels. After receiving magnesium injections, the subjects showed dramatic improvement, and had noticeably improved energy levels, reduced pain, and a better emotional state.

So, if you are tired, don't wait for your symptoms to worsen. Instead, take more magnesium, giving your body the essential ingredient it needs to produce and make use of energy.

Chronic Pain

Lack of magnesium can also lead to chronic pain, especially in the muscles. As Dr. Mildred Seelig says, magnesium is "the mineral of motion"; it is the most important substance for your muscles, controlling their capacity to function and relax. Without magnesium, you would not be able to move. Magnesium is important for the proper regulation of your body's nerves and muscle tone, acting as a gatekeeper and overseeing the amount of calcium that enters into nerve cells. Too much calcium inside a nerve cell will overactivate the nerve. Constant overactivation causes the nerves to send too many messages to the muscles. This in turn causes the muscles to overcontract, resulting in muscle tension, spasms, and ultimately muscle pain and fatigue, leaving you feeling weak and drained.

Compounding this problem is the fact that chronic pain is a stressor that causes your body's stores of magnesium to be used at a faster-than-normal rate. Ongoing pain can quickly deplete magnesium stores, making pain even worse. Types of chronic pain caused or exacerbated by lack of magnesium include back, neck, and shoulder pain, arthritis, carpal tunnel syndrome, and pain or injuries to the soft tissues of the body.

Another cause of pain in the body is the excessive release of a neurotransmitter known as acetylcholine. Neurotransmitters, including acetylcholine, are chemicals that allow nerve impulses, or messages, to be passed from one nerve cell (neuron) to another. The release of too much acetylcholine results in the transmittal of pain impulses. Magnesium is well known for its ability to regulate the release of acetylcholine and prevent it from flooding your system.

In sum, because magnesium deficiency can contribute to the causes of chronic pain, magnesium supplementation can significantly relieve or reverse your symptoms.

Fibromyalgia

Fibromyalgia is a syndrome characterized by fatigue, depression, deep and widespread muscle pain, and the presence of tender points, or specific areas of the body that experience intense pain when pressure is applied. Scientists believe that fibromyalgia is caused by oxidative stress, a type of stress placed on cells and tissues by unstable oxygen compounds called free radicals. Because this oxidative stress results in the destruction or impairment of your body's cells, it has been linked to a number of conditions besides fibromyalgia, including cancer, Parkinson's disease, and certain types of coronary heart disease. Researchers now believe that magnesium deficiency can contribute to oxidative stress, and thus to fibromyalgia.

To test this hypothesis, researchers recently observed a group of sixty women with fibromyalgia against a control group of twenty healthy women. The women with fibromyalgia all had lower levels of magnesium compared to the control group, and the severity of their fibromyalgia symptoms correlated with the degree of magnesium deficiency they had. The women were then divided into three groups. The first group was given 300 mg of magnesium citrate orally each day, the second group was given 10 mg of the fibromyalgia drug amitriptyline each day, and the third group was given the 300 mg of magnesium citrate in combination with the 10 mg of amitriptyline each day. After eight weeks, all three groups were reevaluated. Compared to the group that had taken only the amitriptyline, both of the groups that had taken magnesium (either alone or in conjunction with amitriptyline) showed significant improvements in their symptoms, demonstrating a marked decrease in the presence and sensitivity of tender points and a reduction of pain, fatigue, and psychological distress.

One objection to this study is that the amount of magnesium administered to both groups of women was very low. If the daily dosage of magnesium had been higher, it's likely that the improvements would have been greater, too. Also, as this study shows, magnesium supplementation by itself can be a powerful tool against fibromyalgia; consistent magnesium intake can make the use of drugs like amitriptyline unnecessary.

Headache and Migraine

We're all familiar with headaches—pain or discomfort in the head or neck areas. Headaches and their more severe variant, migraines, can be caused by a variety of factors, including mental or emotional stress, food allergies, exposure to environmental toxins, muscle tension (particularly in the head, shoulders, upper back, and neck, which can constrict blood flow to the brain), skeletal misalignments, and eye strain.

Another significant cause of both headache and migraine is nutritional deficiency, including suboptimal levels of magnesium. Through their research, the director of the New York Headache Center, Dr. Alexander Mauskop, and his colleagues, have shown that people who suffer from migraine and many other types of headache consistently demonstrate a lack of magnesium.

Accordingly, magnesium supplementation can help to prevent headache and migraine in a variety of ways. As you learned in Chapter 4, magnesium relaxes blood vessels and allows them to dilate, reducing spasms and constrictions that can cause headache and migraine. And, as pointed out earlier in this chapter, magnesium regulates the action of your brain's neurotransmitters, which, when unbalanced, can also contribute to headache and migraine by overactivating your nerve cells. Magnesium also helps keep inflammation in check and relaxes head, back, neck, and shoulder muscle tension, all of which can cause or contribute to head pain.

In a study led by Dr. Mauskop, a group of 3,000 migraine patients were given a daily oral supplement of 200 mg of magnesium. This low dose of magnesium was enough to reduce the patients' migraine symptoms by 80 percent. Various other studies have also demonstrated the benefits magnesium has for preventing and relieving headache and migraine symptoms, both by itself and in tandem with other nutrients, especially B vitamins.

Gastrointestinal Problems

Your gastrointestinal (GI) tract, which begins at your mouth and continues down through your esophagus, stomach, and intestines, performs three tasks: it digests the foods you eat, metabolizes the foods so that the nutrients they contain can be properly absorbed, and then eliminates the waste byproducts. All three of these functions are vital to optimal health. When your GI function is impaired, your body is unable to properly absorb and utilize nutrients—including magnesium—from either food or oral supplements.

The result is a vicious cycle of illness, as magnesium deficiency can also *cause* significant gastrointestinal disorders. One of the most common GI disorders associated with a lack of magnesium is constipation, or difficult or infrequent bowel movements. Consequently, people who suffer from chronic constipation should increase their intake of magnesium. Magnesium supplementation has inadvertently been prescribed for years by doctors who tell their patients to add more fiber-rich foods to their daily diet. Fiber-rich foods also tend to be good sources of magnesium, thus doubly helping to improve digestion, and to prevent and reverse constipation.

Magnesium plays an important role in preventing leaky gut syndrome. It also prevents GI tract inflammation, a condition that not only prevents your body from absorbing and metabolizing nutrients, but also destroys or damages immunoglobulin A (IgA), a disease-fighting antibody contained in the protective coating of the GI tract. When your IgA is impaired, your body loses some of its ability to ward off microorganisms that are otherwise held in check within the GI tract, including gut bacteria. This can result in systemic yeast overgrowth, otherwise known as candidiasis. When excess yeast bacteria passes out of the lower GI tract (where it belongs) and into the bloodstream, it acts as a poison, creating havoc for your immune system and potentially triggering the development of other conditions, including allergies, anxiety and depression, chronic fatigue, impaired cognitive and memory function, sexual dysfunction, hyperactivity, hives and other skin problems, respiratory problems, and weight gain, as well as various other GI disorders.

GI disorders rank among the most common chronic health complaints suffered by Americans today. Left unchecked, both leaky gut syndrome and GI tract inflammation can lead to a range of other gastrointestinal conditions, including gastritis (inflammation of the stomach), colitis, Crohn's disease, and irritable bowel syndrome (IBS). All of these conditions can be prevented by magnesium in combination with a healthy diet. Research also indicates that magnesium supplementation can also help reverse these conditions and improve their symptoms.

Heavy Metal Toxicity

Given the prevalence of environmental pollutants in our air, water, and soil supplies, as well as the use of a wide variety of potentially toxic chemicals in industries ranging from agriculture to manufacturing, it is hardly surprising that most Americans host hundreds of different toxins inside their bodies. Consequently, our bodies' organs of detoxification—particularly the liver—are forced to work harder in their attempts to eliminate, or at least minimize the effects of, such toxins. Long-term or intense exposure to heavy metals can produce a variety of health issues, including gastrointestinal dysfunction, organ failure, cancer, and neurological disorders—and can occasionally lead to death.

Magnesium supports your body's detoxification system by allowing the production and proper function of the antioxidants that help you filter out heavy metals. First, discussed in Chapter 4, magnesium plays an essential role in both producing and activating ATP. Without enough ATP, your body lacks the energy it requires to detoxify. Second, magnesium stimulates the sodium-potassium pump of the cellular wall, which regulates the levels of potassium and sodium inside and outside of the cell. When these levels are maintained in their proper ratio (thanks to magnesium) your cells are able to cleanse themselves of wastes, including toxins. In addition, magnesium prevents the influx of excess calcium inside the cells, thus also helping to prevent cellular calcification and premature cell aging and cell death.

Research has shown that magnesium assists in protecting your body from harmful heavy metals, especially aluminum, cadmium, lead, mercury, and nickel. Magnesium helps your liver produce an amino acid called glutathione, a powerful antioxidant that is one of your body's primary weapons against heavy metals. When you are exposed to heavy metals—such as mercury emitted from the placement of dental amalgams, lead in paints, or aluminum contained in vaccines or deodorants—the body instinctively engages glutathione to rid the body of this perceived threat. Once glutathione has been produced, magnesium also keeps it supplied with fuel, allowing for the constant supplies of ATP that glutathione needs in order to carry out the energy-intensive process of detoxification. Without magnesium, your body cannot detoxify itself, and heavy metals and other toxins can build up, damaging cells and tissues and resulting in the health issues mentioned above.

Kidney Stones

Kidney stones are small, hard mineral deposits that form inside the kidneys or within the urinary tract. Approximately one million Americans develop kidney stones each year. Among those that do, between 70 and 80 percent will experience a recurrence of kidney stones later in life. Chronic dehydration is the primary cause of most cases of kidney stone formation, but poor diet (especially a diet high in acidifying foods such as dairy, meats, and starchy carbohydrates) can also be a cause. Genetic predisposition or family history can also be a factor, as can kidney disease and imbalances in the parathyroid gland.

There are four classes of kidney stones, with the most common (80 percent of all cases) being calcium stones. Calcium stones are formed by crystallized deposits of calcium oxalate, a compound that is found in a number of foods, including dark leafy green vegetables, peanuts, and chocolate. People who are prone to kidney stone formation are advised to avoid these foods and increase their intake of pure, filtered water in place of soda, alcohol, coffee, and caffeinated teas, all of which dehydrate the body.

In addition to these dietary measures, people who are at risk for developing calcium stones are also advised to increase their intake of calcium oxalate crystal growth inhibitors—substances that prevent the development of stones. Chief among these inhibitors are citrate (citric acid), vitamin B_6, and magnesium. While you can thus prevent kidney stones by drinking or eating citrus fruits, doctors advise against using magnesium- and B_6-dense foods in a similar manner, as these foods tend to be rich in oxalates—the source of the problem—as well.

Having read this far, you should not be surprised that magnesium is a powerful agent for preventing kidney stones; this book has already documented its capacity to regulate calcium. The use of magnesium in treating and preventing kidney stones was recognized as early as the seventeenth century, and more recent research has validated magnesium's effectiveness as well. In one notable study, fifty-five test subjects with a history of recurring kidney stones were given an oral magnesium supplement at a dose of 500 mg per day, while a control group of forty-three subjects with a history of kidney stone formation took nothing. The patients were followed for up to four years. By the end of the study, there was a 90 percent drop in the rate of kidney stone recurrence among the test subjects who took the magnesium supplements, and 85 percent of the subjects remained stone-free overall. By contrast, 59 percent of the patients in the control group developed new stones.

Research has shown that while B_6 is effective for regulating your liver's production of oxalate, when taken in combination with magnesium, B$_6$ can significantly reduce the risk of kidney stone formation. As you will read in Chapter 6, B$_6$ is a cofactor for magnesium, helping to increase the availability and activation of our favorite mineral and allowing it to inhibit crystal growth. The symbiotic relationship between magnesium and B$_6$ has been known since at least 1974, when a landmark study involving 149 test subjects with a history of recurrent kidney stones showed that patients who were given a combination of magnesium and B$_6$ saw their stone production fall 92 percent, from an average 1.3 stones per person per year to just 0.1.

Osteoporosis

Osteoporosis is a condition characterized by thin, brittle, porous bones. It affects nearly 16 percent of all postmenopausal women in the United States. Four percent of older American men also suffer from osteoporosis. Overall, osteoporosis accounts for over two million bone fractures each and every year, primarily of the hips, spine or wrist.

American statistics contrast sharply with those of traditional cultures, where osteoporosis and other chronic degenerative health conditions are virtually unknown. As clinical nutritionist and medical anthropologist Dr. Susan Brown has shown, the difference can be attributed to diet: Compared with the standard American diet, which features acidifying foods and beverages (refined carbohydrates, sugar, excessive animal proteins, sodas, and juices), traditional diets tend to feature alkalizing foods. Such foods act to maintain proper pH balance, preventing the development and buildup of acids, which are proven to set the stage for disease. Additionally, many of the alkaline foods found within such diets are rich in minerals, including magnesium.

Based on the research of Dr. Brown and others, it is obvious that shifting to a healthier, more alkalizing diet is an essential step for both preventing and helping to reverse osteoporosis. Certain nutritional supplements, including magnesium, can also provide significant benefits. Research indicates that magnesium not only helps to maintain and even restore bone density, but also improves calcium's ability to improve bone health by regulating the metabolism and deployment of calcium in the body. Magnesium also plays a similar role for vitamin D, another essential vitamin in maintaining bone health.

Various studies have demonstrated magnesium's ability to maintain and restore bone density. In one such study, 75 percent of postmenopausal women who took a daily oral magnesium supplement for two years saw their bone mineral density increase by 1 to 8 percent. This result is all the more noteworthy because postmenopausal women typically lose bone density at a rate of 3 to 8 percent each year. These findings were confirmed by a larger study of over 2,000 elderly men and women, which revealed that increased magnesium intake from both diet and supplementation resulted in improved total-body bone density in white men and women, although the same benefits were not observed in black men and women, who have naturally lower osteoporosis rates.

Premenstrual Syndrome (PMS)

Premenstrual syndrome (PMS) encompasses a range of physical symptoms—including bloating, breast tenderness, joint pain, fatigue, headache, fluid retention—and emotional or behavioral issues, including mood swings, irritability, depression, anxiety, bouts of crying, and appetite changes or food cravings.PMS affects an estimated 70 to 90 percent of women prior to their monthly menstrual cycle, with up to 40 percent of women experiencing severe symptoms.

Studies have shown that women who suffer from PMS typically have low levels of magnesium in their red blood cells. In one such study, researchers from the Universities of Modena and Pavia in Italy found that women who took 360 mg of magnesium each day from the fifteenth day of their menstrual cycle to the beginning of their next period all reported noticeably lessened PMS symptoms when compared to the control group, who took no magnesium and whose symptoms remained unchanged.

In another study conducted by researchers at the University of Reading in England, similar results were achieved with only

200 mg of magnesium. This study found that magnesium reduced PMS-related symptoms of fluid retention, breast tenderness and bloating by 40 percent, while also significantly reducing PMS-induced weight gain and swelling in the participants' hands and legs.

The research shows that magnesium works to relieve PMS symptoms by acting as a muscle relaxant, reducing cramping and preventing blood vessels from tensing or spasming, thus also alleviating or preventing PMS-related headaches and migraines. Because the stress associated with PMS can deplete the body of its magnesium stores, magnesium supplementation can help relieve emotional and behavioral symptoms, including anxiety, depression, irritability, tension, and appetite changes. Magnesium also serves to replenish diminished energy supplies, and has a diuretic effect, helping to ease fluid retention and bloating.

Sleep Disorders

According to the National Sleep Foundation, approximately 60 percent of all Americans suffer from insomnia or other sleep-related problems. Sleep is a critical time for your body to rest and repair itself—hormones regulating growth and metabolism are released, muscles are repaired, and memories are consolidated. When sleep is disrupted, your body suffers; studies have repeatedly shown links between sleep disorders and a number of other unhealthy conditions, including depression, obesity, and cardiovascular disease.

While there are many causes of sleep disorders, stress is one of the most significant and controllable factors. Stress affects sleep by disrupting your body's circadian rhythms, which are a series of physical, mental, and behavioral changes that occur over a twenty-four-hour cycle, largely as a result of varying levels of light and darkness. Sleepiness, body temperature, and hormone concentrations all fluctuate throughout the day according to circadian rhythms.

Among the substances whose concentrations are subject to circadian rhythms is the stress hormone cortisol. When the sun rises, your body begins to ramp up its production of hormones that induce wakefulness, including cortisol. Under normal, healthy conditions, your body's natural cortisol concentration reaches its peak between 8AM and 9AM, telling your body to wake up and get work done. From that point on, your cortisol level drops progressively, reaching its lowest point at midnight, when, deprived of this "go" hormone, you finally nod off. About two hours later, your body once more begins to produce cortisol, gradually increasing production until it peaks and you wake again. When this cycle unfolds the way nature intended, your waking hours are productive and your sleep is deep and restful.

Unfortunately, the normal ebb and flow of cortisol is easily disrupted by stress. As discussed in Chapter 2, stress forces your body to produce more cortisol on a regular basis in order to deal with the pressures of daily life. As anybody who has experienced stress can attest, this can have serious consequences for your ability to sleep. Sometimes stress can even cause the cortisol cycle to reverse itself, with your cortisol level peaking during normal sleeping time and reaching its lowest point upon awakening. Flooded with cortisol at the wrong time, you're anxious and alert when you should be sleeping, and groggy and tired when you should be energized. Worse still, this disruption of cortisol's normal cycle is in and of itself another systemic stressor, further contributing to your body's magnesium depletion.

Stress also disrupts another hormone that is implicated in the circadian sleep cycle, melatonin. Melatonin complements cortisol; it is a hormone that encourages sleep, as cortisol encourages wakefulness. As your cortisol level drops throughout the day, your melatonin level rises, peaking at midnight and helping you nod off. After that point, melatonin production decreases, and then stops completely when the sun begins to rise, signaling your body to produce wakeful hormones like cortisol so that you can get up and go about your daily business. There are four different steps that your body takes to metabolize melatonin and make it usable, and all four of these steps require the presence of magnesium. Under periods of prolonged stress, you become magnesium deficient, and thus can't make the melatonin you need to get to sleep at night.

As you can see, without magnesium, your body simply can't produce or regulate the hormones that allow it to carry out its natural sleep cycle. Thus difficulty sleeping is often yet another effect of magnesium deficiency. While doctors often recommend that people with sleep disorders or insomnia take melatonin in order to reset their circadian rhythms, it makes more sense to treat the root of the problem—lack of magnesium. Instead of relying on melatonin supplements or sleeping pills, both of which carry risks, it is far easier to remedy your sleeping problems by increasing your daily intake of magnesium. This fact is borne out by scientific research.

One study involved 100 men and women between the ages of 51 and 85, all of whom suffered from poor-quality sleep. Half the group was given a daily magnesium supplement of 320 mg, while the other half was given a placebo. At the end of the study, researchers found that the participants in the magnesium group not only experienced improved sleep, but also had lower levels of chronic inflammation, another stressor linked to poor sleep.

Research has also confirmed that magnesium supplementation increases deep levels of sleep, regulates brain wave patterns and improves abnormal brain wave patterns associated with insomnia, and reduces the amount of time it takes to fall asleep. In addition, magnesium has been shown to help symptoms of sleep apnea and restless leg syndrome.

CONCLUSION

While the primary goal of this book is to make you aware of the significance of magnesium in maintaining heart health and preventing heart disease, this chapter demonstrates that magnesium can have direct benefits for countless other common diseases and conditions. Moreover, it's important to point out that many of these health issues are related, both to each other and to cardiovascular disease. For example, chronic fatigue syndrome can have symptoms of muscle pain and headache, and can lead to depression; chronic sleep deprivation is a risk factor for mental disorders, obesity, high blood pressure, and also heart attack. This cross-correlation between conditions is not coincidental: Magnesium deficiency underlies most, if not all, of these health problems.

Thus, an understanding of magnesium can not only help you treat these serious health issues, but also prevent their very occurrence. In addition, by using magnesium to forestall the onset of a specific condition, you may very well be allowing your body to fight off other conditions that are associated with it, including heart disease. When taken appropriately, magnesium can—and should—be a powerful weapon in your fight for a better, healthier life.

Now that you have read this far, the time has come to put the information you have just read into practice. Chapter 6 will teach you how to determine your body's own magnesium levels, and also how to most effectively ensure that you are meeting your body's daily magnesium needs through both proper diet and magnesium supplementation. Read on!

6

How to Take Magnesium

Now that you understand the importance of magnesium for your heart and overall health, it's time to discuss what you can do to ensure that you get all the magnesium that your body needs on a daily basis. This chapter tells you everything you need to know about optimizing your magnesium levels. In it, you will learn how to evaluate your current magnesium status and needs—and, accordingly, how to increase that status through diet, supplements, and other methods. You will also find information on the various types of magnesium and the precautions you should take when consuming magnesium. Finally, you will learn how to monitor and maintain your magnesium levels, so that you will always enjoy the good health that this magnificent nutrient can provide.

DETERMINING YOUR CURRENT MAGNESIUM STATUS

Despite the mountain of evidence pointing to magnesium as an important component of overall health, there still remains a great divide between what we know and how we use this information. At this time, most doctors do not routinely screen their patients for magnesium deficiency, though this will surely change as the dangers of this condition become better known and understood. In addition, the standard blood panel—the set of blood tests that serves as the best indicator of what's going on inside our bodies—does not usually evaluate magnesium levels, and those that do often use an inaccurate form of measurement. In order to determine your current magnesium status, you are going to have to be proactive.

The first step is to find a physician who will be able to guide you on your journey to better health. Preferably, you will find a doctor who is trained in integrative medicine, or one whose treatment methods emphasize diet and nutrition over pharmaceuticals. To help you out, there is a list of organizations whose memberships comprise nutritionally oriented physicians in the Resources section of this book.

Blood Testing

Next, you should evaluate your body's current magnesium status by having your doctor order a magnesium red blood cell (RBC-Mg) blood test. You can get this test done even if you don't have a doctor—a number of medical laboratories now operate independently, allowing you to buy medical tests online without a prescription. You visit their website, select the test you want to have done, and the company will direct you to a nearby facility that will perform the test. Typically, your results will be emailed to you within seventy-two hours from the time that your blood is drawn. Please note that at this time, the RBC-Mg test is not available by mail to residents of Maryland, Massachusetts, New Jersey, New York, or Rhode Island. If you live in these states, you will still be able to obtain the test through your physician.

It is important that you order a magnesium red blood cell test, and not the more widely available serum magnesium test. Because the RBC-Mg test measures the amount of magnesium that is in your red blood cells, it is a far more accurate measure of your magnesium levels than the serum test, which simply evaluates the amount of free magnesium in your plasma.

Currently, the normal reference range for the RBC-Mg levels is 4.2 to 6.8 mg/dL Prior to 1963, however, normal levels were said to range from 5.0 to 7.0 mg/dL. The change essentially lowers the bar for an American population that is overwhelmingly magnesium deficient; by reducing the reference range, more Americans can be considered to have a "normal" magnesium status. The earlier reference range is more realistic. Because "normal" levels of magnesium are not necessarily optimal levels, it is best to consider any RBC-Mg reading under 5.5 mg/dL to be a clear indication of magnesium deficiency.

ASSESSING YOUR MAGNESIUM NEEDS

Knowing your body's magnesium status is the first step you can take towards better health. But how can you remedy a deficiency or help maintain optimal levels? This section shows you how to determine the amount of magnesium your body needs in order to perform at its best.

The Institute of Medicine of the National Academy of Sciences recommends the following dietary reference intakes (DRIs):

DRIs FOR CHILDREN AND TEENAGERS	
AGES	**DOSAGE**
Ages 1 to 3	40 to 80 mg/day
Ages 4 to 8	130 mg/day
Ages 9 to 13	240 mg/day
Males, ages 14 to 18	410 mg/day
Females, ages 14 to 18	360 mg/day

(**Note:** Children should not take magnesium supplements without a doctor's supervision.)

DRIs FOR ADULTS	
AGES	**DOSAGE**
Males, ages 19 to 30	400 mg/day
Males, age 31 and over	420 mg/day
Females, ages 19 to 30	310 mg/day

DRIs for Adults *(cont.)*	
Ages	**Dosage**
Females, age 31 and over	320 mg/day
Pregnant females, ages 19 to 30	350 mg/day
Pregnant females, age 31 and over	360 mg/day
Breastfeeding females, ages 19 to 30	310 mg/day
Breastfeeding females, age 31 and over	320 mg/day

The DRIs are problematic because they measure only the smallest amounts of each nutrient needed to achieve minimum health, not the amounts that are necessary to create and maintain optimal health. As this book has pointed out, nearly all Americans today are deficient in magnesium, and the dietary reference intake levels suggested are not high enough to correct this problem. The DRIs also fail to take into account the fact that your magnesium needs change depending on the varieties and levels of stressors in your life.

Because the DRIs are thus inadequate, another set of guidelines must be used. Your magnesium burn rate, or MBR, evaluates your daily exposure to stress. The more stress you are under, the more magnesium your body burns. Your MBR is the metabolic price tag for all the pressure and tension that stress causes.

To determine your MBR, appraise how often you are exposed to each of the stressors we listed in Chapter 2. Be honest with yourself. How many stressors do you encounter on a daily basis, and how intensely do you experience them? To help you along in this process, answer the questions as truthfully as you can.

It is easy to determine your magnesium burn rate. To help you out, the questionnaire on the following two pages will allow you to appraise how often you are exposed to each of the stressors discussed in Chapter 2. Be honest with yourself—only then will you be able to get an accurate picture of how quickly stress causes you to use up your magnesium stores.

How Stressed Are You?

Consider social stressors:	Yes	No	Unsure
1. Do you have a hard time handling mental or emotional stress?	☐	☐	☐
2. Do you have stress at work?	☐	☐	☐
3. Do you have stress at home?	☐	☐	☐
4. Do you have stress from personal relationships?	☐	☐	☐
5. Do you experience these stressors on a daily basis?	☐	☐	☐
6. Do you experience these stressors on an hourly basis?	☐	☐	☐

Consider physiological stressors:	Yes	No	Unsure
7. Are you recovering from surgery?	☐	☐	☐
8. Do you exercise frequently and/or at a high level of intensity?	☐	☐	☐
9. Do you suffer from arthritis and/or damaged tissues?	☐	☐	☐
10. Do you suffer from cardiovascular disease, particularly hypertension?	☐	☐	☐
11. Do you suffer from chronic pain?	☐	☐	☐
12. Do you suffer from diabetes?	☐	☐	☐
13. Do you suffer from elevated cholesterol and/or triglyceride levels?	☐	☐	☐
14. Do you suffer from insomnia or other sleep disorders?	☐	☐	☐
15. Do you suffer from migraine headaches?	☐	☐	☐

Consider dietary stressors: Yes   No   Unsure

16. Do you habitually eat a lot of processed foods? ☐ ☐ ☐

17. Do you habitually drink acid-forming beverages, such as soda, coffee, and alcohol? ☐ ☐ ☐

18. Do you eat out regularly? ☐ ☐ ☐

19. Do you follow a high- or low-protein diet? ☐ ☐ ☐

20. Do you follow a high-carbohydrate diet? ☐ ☐ ☐

21. Does your diet emphasize caloric restriction? ☐ ☐ ☐

22. Do you take calcium or vitamin D supplements? ☐ ☐ ☐

23. Do you suffer from chronic diarrhea or other gastrointestinal problems? ☐ ☐ ☐

Consider environmental stressors: Yes   No   Unsure

24. Are you exposed to hot weather for long periods of time? ☐ ☐ ☐

25. Are you regularly exposed to toxins such as heavy metals? ☐ ☐ ☐

26. Are you exposed to polluted air/smog at home and/or your workplace? ☐ ☐ ☐

27. Do you use pharmaceutical drugs (see the list on pages 61 to 63) on a regular basis? ☐ ☐ ☐

TOTALS   ____   ____   ____

How many times did you answer "yes"? The more "yes" answers you had, the more stressors you face, and the higher your MBR will be. And the higher your MBR is, the more magnesium you need.

While there is no such thing as a one-size-fits-all daily allowance for magnesium, a good rule of thumb is to take about three milligrams of magnesium for every pound of body weight at the minimum. This formula is based on the one developed by Dr. Mildred Seeling, the scientist you read about in Chapter 4. For example, under normal circumstances, a woman weighing 120 pounds should take at least 360 mg of magnesium, while a 200-pound man would take 600 mg. Under more stressful circumstances, you'll need to increase your dosage—Dr. Seelig recommends raising your magnesium intake to five milligrams for every pound of body weight. This means that if confronted with a particularly difficult workweek or emotional crisis, our 120-pound woman might take 600 mg of magnesium, and our 200-pound man would take about 1,000 mg—far more than the DRIs would suggest.

The following chart will help you calculate your magnesium needs based on your weight. Magnesium intake levels are presented as a range of values, to allow you to account for variations in your daily stress levels. If you are having a particularly stressful day and your magnesium burn rate is higher, you may want to increase your dosage to reflect the upper part of the range for your weight class. Or you can simply add 100 to 200 mg of magnesium to your normal daily magnesium intake to help your body cope with the greater stress burden.

OPTIMAL DAILY MAGNESIUM INTAKE REFERENCE	
WEIGHT (POUNDS)	**MAGNESIUM RANGE (MILLIGRAMS)**
75–100	250–500
100–125	300–650
125–150	400–750
150–175	450–900
175–200	550–1,000
200–250	600–1,200
250+	750–1,250

Once you've figured out approximately how much magnesium you need, it's time to consider how best to get it.

GETTING MAGNESIUM FROM YOUR DIET

A wholesome, well-balanced diet is the key to good health. Consequently, in order to supplement your magnesium intake, you should first look to increase your consumption of foods that are rich in this nutrient. As explained in Chapter 2, magnesium is a key component of chlorophyll. So it shouldn't surprise you that chlorophyll-rich green vegetables are good sources of magnesium, especially Swiss chard, collard greens, mustard greens, beet greens, kale, parsley, spinach, asparagus, and broccoli.

But a food source doesn't have to be green in order to possess high concentrations of magnesium—nuts, legumes (beans), and dried fruit are also excellent sources. The list on the following page of magnesium-rich foods is derived from the United States Department of Agriculture's National Nutrient Database. To the right of each food is the quantity of magnesium present in a 100-gram (3.5-oz) serving of that food.

Various seeds are also loaded in magnesium: flaxseed (10 mg per tsp), pumpkin seed (74 mg per oz), sesame seed (32 mg per tsp), and sunflower seeds (37 mg per oz). So are certain spices, including coriander powder (6 mg per tsp), cumin (8 mg per tsp), fennel seed (8 mg per tsp), and dried parsley (6 mg per tsp). Small servings of these seeds and spices can go a long way toward improving your magnesium status—if considered in terms of 100-gram servings, the magnesium content of these foods would actually exceed many of those listed on the following page.

SUPPLEMENTING WITH MAGNESIUM

While any attempt to optimize your magnesium level should begin with your diet, there are a number of factors that make it difficult to meet all your magnesium needs through food sources alone. As shown in Chapter 2, magnesium levels in food can vary from region to region and day to day, due to conditions that impair the

The Magnesium in Your Food*

- Rice bran—781 mg
- Wheat bran—611 mg
- Cocoa powder—499 mg
- Brazil nuts—376 mg
- Almonds—268 mg
- Cashews—260 mg
- Blackstrap molasses—242 mg
- Peanuts—176 mg
- Hazelnuts—163 mg
- Walnuts—158 mg
- Pecans—132 mg
- Kelp—121 mg
- Coconut (dried)—90 mg
- Spinach (cooked) –88 mg
- Swiss chard (cooked)—86 mg
- Lima beans—74 mg
- Beet greens (cooked)—68 mg
- Figs (dried)—68 mg
- Quinoa—64 mg
- Tuna (fresh, cooked)—64 mg
- Soybeans (cooked)—60 mg
- Crab (cooked)—58 mg
- Dates—54 mg
- Navy beans—53 mg
- Parsley—50 mg
- Pinto beans—50 mg
- Kale (raw) —47 mg

- Kidney beans—45 mg
- Millet—44 mg
- Brown rice (long-grained)—43 mg
- Chives—42 mg
- Prunes (dried)—41 mg
- Green peas (cooked)—39 mg
- Shrimp—39 mg
- Salmon—37 mg
- Scallops—37 mg
- Raisins—32 mg
- Avocado (Hass)—29 mg
- Cheddar cheese—28 mg
- Halibut—28 mg
- Banana—27 mg
- Sweet potato (baked)—27 mg
- Beets (cooked)—23 mg
- Barley—22 mg
- Broccoli (cooked)—21 mg
- Collard greens—21 mg
- Shallots—21 mg
- Cauliflower (raw)—15 mg
- Asparagus—14 mg
- Leeks—14 mg
- Mustard greens—13 mg
- Onions (cooked)—11 mg
- Tomatoes—11 mg

* *Based on 100 gram (3.5 oz) portions.*

general nutrient density of our agricultural products. In addition, magnesium absorption can be limited by impaired digestion, improper cooking methods, interactions with other food-based chemical compounds, low- or high-protein diets, acid-forming foods, and pharmaceutical drugs. Accordingly, you should reinforce and increase your magnesium intake with supplements.

It is important that you have all the information you need before beginning any magnesium supplementation regimen. As with any health initiative, it is advisable that you consult with a physician, who will be able to give you specific advice based on your medical history and current health condition. At the very least, you should make sure to determine your magnesium status with an RBC-Mg test and assess your magnesium burn rate. Once you have this information, you and your doctor will be able to come up with an appropriate plan for magnesium supplementation.

The Various Forms of Magnesium

Choosing a magnesium supplement can be a very confusing business. Magnesium supplements come in many forms and can be taken either internally and externally. Dosages vary from form to form and brand to brand—although nearly all magnesium supplements are measured in milligrams, with amounts ranging from 100 mg to 500 mg. Chemical composition can also differ: Some brands use only one type of magnesium compound, while others mix types, and still others include non-magnesium ingredients such as calcium, folate, and other vitamins. Not all forms of magnesium are alike; thus the benefits they offer can vary. The following guide will help you figure out the best supplement for your needs, detailing the many forms of magnesium and their different applications and benefits.

Oral Magnesium Supplements

Magnesium supplements are most commonly found in forms that can be taken orally—tablets, capsules, powders, and liquids. Tablets are coated with sugar or a similar substance, preventing their magnesium from being absorbed into the bloodstream immediately; their primary advantage is that they can be cut in half (or even into thirds) if a specific dosage is desired. Capsules are coated in gelatin that dissolves upon contact with liquid; they are more easily swallowed and their contents more quickly absorbed, though they can't be subdivided the way tablets can be. Powders are useful for people who have difficulty swallowing pills; the prescribed dosage is simply mixed into a volume of water and drunk. Magnesium also comes in liquid form, often as milk of magnesia—but this medium is poorly absorbed by the intestine and is primarily used for its laxative effect (see below).

Types of Magnesium Supplements and Their Uses

By and large, any magnesium supplement can provide benefits, but certain forms of magnesium can have special benefits for specific health complaints. Here is a breakdown of the various uses of these different forms of magnesium.

General Use: Magnesium chloride (applied directly to the skin or used in a foot bath), magnesium glycinate, magnesium malate.

Brain Health: Nearly all forms of magnesium cross the blood-brain barrier to benefit the brain. Magnesium orotate and magnesium l-threonate are especially useful in this regard.

Gastrointestinal Health: Magnesium citrate and magnesium lactate. Milk of magnesia (liquid magnesium oxide) is frequently used for constipation.

Heart Health: Magnesium malate, magnesium taurate.

Joint and Muscle Health: Most oral forms of magnesium help prevent and remedy joint and muscle pain. Topical applications of magnesium oil and Epsom salt baths are also excellent for relieving joint and muscle pain.

It's also possible to buy concentrated magnesium drops at your local health store; these, too, can be added to your drinking water each day.

While any magnesium supplementation is better than none, for convenience, ease of application, precision of dosage, and widespread availability, I recommend using either tablets or capsules in order to supplement your magnesium intake. That said, there are still a number of different factors to consider when choosing a magnesium pill.

Bioavailability

As discussed earlier, your body doesn't necessarily receive all of the nutrients contained in a serving of food or a supplement. Various factors affect your ability to absorb these different nutrients. The term that is used to describe this relative absorption rate is bioavailability, or the amount of a nutrient or drug that can be readily taken into your bloodstream from your digestive system at a given time. Certain forms of magnesium—such as magnesium malate, magnesium glycinate, and magnesium taurate—are more bioavailable, and thus recommended by most healthcare practitioners. Unfortunately, the forms of magnesium most commonly used in oral magnesium supplements—magnesium oxide and magnesium chloride—are less bioavailable, and thus have a lower absorption rate. These forms are more likely to pass through your digestive system without being absorbed into your bloodstream.

In choosing a magnesium supplement, consult the ingredient list to ensure that the form of magnesium used is one of the more readily absorbed compounds recommended above. When using topical or transdermal forms of magnesium, concerns about bioavailability are lessened because the magnesium is absorbed directly through your skin.

Timed Release

It's important to consider not only the chemical bioavailability of oral magnesium supplements, but also your body's physical ability to absorb them over time. Some oral forms of magnesium pass through your system quickly because your body is unable to absorb all the magnesium at once. As a result, these forms can cause loose bowels even at low doses, since your body gets rid of whatever it can't use at the time. (In fact, it is this bowel-loosening effect that has made milk of magnesia famous as a treatment for constipation.) This is particularly unfortunate, since diarrhea, or loose bowels, can make a magnesium deficiency worse. Instead, choose forms of magnesium that have timed release—sometimes called extended or sustained release. These forms slowly discharge their magnesium over a period of hours, improving the likelihood that your body will be able to absorb as much of the nutrient as it needs and greatly reducing the risk of laxative effects and digestive discomfort.

Cofactors

To maximize your magnesium absorption, you should be sure to take vitamin B_6 along with your magnesium supplement. Vitamin B_6 is a cofactor for magnesium and enhances its bioavailability, allowing you to get the most out of this important nutrient. Try to take the active form of B_6, known as pyridoxal-5´-phosphate, or P-5-P, which can be used by the body immediately.

When to Take Supplements

Once you have determined your total daily supplement intake, divide that dose into increments of two or three—whichever works out best in terms of the specific magnesium dosage of the pills you've bought. Take your supplement with food, at mealtime (breakfast, lunch, and/or dinner), or at evenly spaced intervals throughout the day. For example, if you are supposed to take 600 mg each day, and you've bought 200-mg pills, you can take one pill at each of your meals. Although magnesium is generally beneficial to sleep disorders, because of its role in producing energy, magnesium can sometimes interfere with sleep. Until you rule out this problem, you may want to take your last dose of magnesium no later than 5 or 6PM each day. Should you experience loose bowels or stomach upset when using magnesium supplements, try reducing your total daily dose temporarily, then build it back up as your tolerance increases. You may also benefit from using a timed release formulation. If symptoms continue, stop your supplementation and consult with a physician to determine whether you have any underlying gastrointestinal problems.

Transdermal Magnesium Supplements

While pills and other oral supplements offer convenience and precise doses, there are other advantages to forms of magnesium that can be absorbed transdermally, or through the skin. These methods can be useful for people who prefer not to take pills, or for people who are interested in reaping the additional benefits that transdermal applications have to offer.

Magnesium Oil

Magnesium oil is not actually an oil at all, but rather a highly concentrated suspension of magnesium chloride in water. It is meant for topical applications only, and should not be taken internally. Instead, magnesium oil can be rubbed directly onto your skin, where it is absorbed and immediately transmitted into your bloodstream, which will transport this magnesium compound to your tissues and cells. For best results, apply the oil to your chest, abdomen, arms, or legs, and allow it to dry fully, maximizing absorption. Then wash off any residue that remains. Magnesium oil is useful not only for increasing your general magnesium intake, but also for remedying superficial cuts and scarring.

You can also use magnesium oil to create a restorative footbath, adding one or two ounces to enough hot water to cover both of your feet in a tub or soaking pan. Simply soak your feet until the water cools, which usually takes about twenty minutes. There is no need to air-dry your feet, as with the magnesium oil above; you will have gotten all the magnesium you need during the soak itself. Ideally, you should do magnesium oil rubs or footbaths once a day, or at least three times a week.

Epsom Salt Baths

Epsom salt baths are another excellent way to obtain more magnesium, while also soothing muscle aches and pains. Epsom salt is made up of a form of magnesium called magnesium sulfate, and is readily available at just about every local drugstore in the nation. To prepare an Epsom salt bath, simply add one to two cups of Epsom salt to a bathtub filled with warm water, along with one cup of baking soda (*not* baking powder). Then enter the bathtub and soak your body for thirty to forty minutes. For best results, try taking at least one Epsom salt bath each week.

It is difficult to quantify the exact amounts of magnesium you will receive from these transdermal applications, but the results will speak for themselves. By adding magnesium oil and Epsom salt baths to your supplementation regimen, you will not only help to optimize your magnesium intake, but you will also obtain a variety of other benefits for your skin, muscles, and overall stress levels.

Cautions and Contraindications

Although magnesium supplements are generally very safe to use, there are a few side effects and precautions to consider when taking magnesium. People with kidney disease should not take magnesium except under a doctor's supervision, because their kidneys may not be able to excrete excess magnesium. Children and the elderly should also avoid using magnesium supplements without doctor supervision.

As mentioned earlier, the most common problems associated with magnesium supplementation are stomach upset and loose bowels, both of which will usually subside quickly after either reducing the magnesium dosage or switching to a better tolerated form of magnesium, such as a timed-release formula.

Other side effects are rare, but can be serious. They include nausea, vomiting, unhealthily low blood pressure levels, confusion, slowed heart rate, respiratory problems, and deficiencies of other minerals. These problems usually develop as a result of extremely high magnesium consumption. If they occur, stop supplementing with magnesium and seek immediate medical help.

Magnesium can also interfere with certain pharmaceutical drugs, and therefore should never be used in supplement form without your doctor's permission and oversight. The specific drugs or classes of drugs for which magnesium may be contraindicated include:

- **Antibiotics:** Magnesium may reduce the absorption of certain classes of antibiotics, including aminoglycosides (Amikin, Garamycin), fluoroquinolones (Cipro, Levaquin), tetracyclines (Tetracycline, Doxycycline), and nitrofurantoins (Macrodantin, Macrobid). Magnesium should therefore be taken one hour before or two hours after taking these medications.

- **Beta blockers:** Magnesium can slow heart beat abnormally and reduce overall cardiac output when taken with this class of drugs, which includes labetalol (Trandate) and atenolol (Tenormin). Magnesium can also interfere with the absorption of beta blockers.

- **Biphosphonates:** Magnesium can interfere with the absorption of osteoporosis drugs, including alendronate (Fosamax) and risedronate (Actonel). For this reason, magnesium supplements should be taken one hour before or two hours after taking these medications.

- **Calcium Channel Blockers:** Magnesium may increase the risk of dizziness, nausea, and fluid retention when used with this class of antihypertensive drugs, which includes nifedipine (Procardia) and amlodipine (Norvasc).

- **Corticosteroids:** Magnesium may increase muscle relaxation and blood clotting when used with this class of drugs, which includes prednisone (Deltasone) and dexamethasone (Decadron). In addition, corticosteroids can deplete magnesium levels.

- **Diabetes Medications:** Magnesium may interfere with the ability of these drugs to control blood sugar levels. Medications include glipizide (Glucotrol) and glyburide (Micronase/ Glynase).

- **Digoxin (Lanoxin):** Low blood levels of magnesium can increase digoxin's side effects, including heart palpitations and nausea. In addition, digoxin can cause more magnesium to be lost in the urine. People taking digoxin may need to take a magnesium supplement, and should have their magnesium levels monitored by their doctor.

Magnesium Supplementation and Safety Issues

When used as directed, mineral supplements pose virtually no safety risks. To reach levels of toxicity (overdose), you would need to ignore our directions and consume massive amounts of minerals for prolonged periods of time. This explains why there are no confirmed records of serious adverse side effects resulting from people taking reasonable doses of magnesium.

While it is thus highly unlikely that you will ever take too much magnesium, there are some issues to take into consideration before beginning a supplementation program. As discussed in Chapter 2, several factors can affect the bioavailability of magnesium—for example, pharmaceutical drugs can limit the absorption of magnesium, while regular exercise can increase it. In addition, magnesium can potentially interact and interfere with the proper functioning of certain drugs (see page 146). People with kidney disease should also avoid magnesium, as their bodies are no longer capable of excreting excess amounts of this mineral.

If you have any doubts about taking magnesium, you should consult your physician, who will take your personal medical history into account and help you determine how much magnesium is right for you.

- **Diuretics:** Like diogoxin, diuretics like furosemide (Lasix) and bumetanide (Bumex) can also deplete magnesium levels, thus requiring magnesium monitoring and the likely use of magnesium supplements.

- **Levothyroxine** (Synthroid, Levothroid): Magnesium may decrease the effectiveness of this drug, which is primarily used to treat hypothyroidism.

- **Penicillamine:** Magnesium can decrease the absorption of this drug, which is used to treat rheumatoid arthritis and Wilson's disease, particularly when high doses are used over a long period of time. In turn, penicillamine can also decrease the absorption of magnesium.

If you are currently using any of these drugs, consult your doctor to determine whether it is still advisable to take magnesium. Most of the time, it is perfectly safe to do so; many drug interactions can be avoided simply by staggering the times you take magnesium and your pharmaceuticals. That said, you should always use caution when beginning any supplementation program. Even if you have no contraindications for magnesium, proceed slowly in the beginning. Start by taking a single dose of magnesium and wait twenty-four hours to make sure you have no adverse reactions. Contact your doctor immediately if any severe reactions do occur.

It's important to note that not only are the above drugs contraindicated for use with magnesium, but many of them also serve to rob your body's existing magnesium stores. In addition, some of these drugs are prescribed to perform tasks that could potentially be done by magnesium itself. For these reasons, you may want to avoid using pharmaceutical drugs if at all possible. Talk to your healthcare provider about the option of using magnesium as an alternative to these drugs; a good doctor will be receptive to the idea. If it is not advisable to use magnesium as an alternative, you may need to boost your intake to account for the deficiency that these pharmaceutical drugs can cause.

MONITORING YOUR PROGRESS

As your supplementation program continues, be sure to monitor your progress. Consult regularly with your physician, and take follow-up RBC-Mg tests every year to keep an eye on your current magnesium status. Doing so will provide you with a clearer understanding of the progress you are making, and will indicate whether you need to adjust your magnesium dosage levels. You may need to periodically reassess your magnesium needs, which will change as the number of stressors in your life increase or decrease.

Keep in mind that magnesium, like all other nutrients, works from the inside out, meaning that its benefits begin at the cellular level and start to become more outwardly apparent once the health of the cells improve. This means that you may not notice any benefits initially. Be patient. Depending on your current health condition, it may be a few months or more before you notice all of the improvements that magnesium provides to your heart and overall cardiovascular system, as well as to your muscles, immune system, nervous system, and other areas of your body.

CONCLUSION

Now that you have read this chapter, you know what you must do to ensure that your body gets all of the magnesium it needs. Start by determining your body's current magnesium status—order an RBC-Mg test and discuss the results with your doctor. Then, objectively evaluate your magnesium burn rate, considering the number of stressors to which you are regularly exposed and appraising their intensity levels.

From there, increase your intake of magnesium-rich foods, including them in every meal; your diet is the foundation upon which your health rests. Then, if necessary—and for the vast majority of people, it will be—add magnesium supplements according to the guidelines and precautions provided here. As you do so, listen to your body, note how you feel, and periodically retest your magnesium status as you go you along.

If you follow these simple steps, magnesium can make a tremendous impact on your health. By being proactive about your magnesium status, you put your health into your own hands. The key is to be consistent about supplementing—and to be patient as you allow magnificent magnesium to go to work for you.

Conclusion

O ver the years, Americans have spent trillions of dollars in order to treat cardiovascular disease with expensive, ineffective, and often dangerous drugs. Yet heart disease continues to be the number one killer in the United States. Why is this? Is it possible that we have failed to locate the true source of the problem? With new research pouring in every day, the evidence has become increasingly clear. As the starved heart model indicates, one potential cause of heart disease is a deep-seated condition whose ill effects extend to every cell in your body—magnesium deficiency. Magnesium deficiency is a major cause of inflammation, which then sets the wheels in motion for the development of atherosclerosis and all its complications—especially heart attacks and strokes.

If you've read this far, you know that there is an easy way to combat this insidious problem—get more magnesium in your life! Research overwhelmingly indicates that you can prevent or protect against most forms of heart disease with the effortless addition of a little magnesium to your daily routine. By increasing your intake of magnesium, you can vastly reduce your risk of heart disease, and even help reduce any conditions you might already have.

The solution is so simple, yet its significance for your health is immense and far-ranging. This humble nutrient can make a huge difference not only for your heart, but for every other major organ system in your body, allowing you to reverse or ward off many other serious conditions, including type 2 diabetes, metabolic syndrome, fibromyalgia, and insomnia.

This book had two main goals. One, to provide you with the information you need to better understand your cardiovascular system and the various types of heart disease. Two, to share with you the most relevant studies that show how magnesium is linked to your heart's health.

But a book is only as good as the lessons you learn from it—and put into action. Having read this book, you've taken the first step toward improving your health. Now it's time to take the next steps! Let's review what you must do to increase your magnesium levels and decrease your risk of heart disease and other conditions.

Begin by reducing or eliminating the factors in your life that contribute to magnesium deficiency. As you'll recall from Chapter 2, a primary cause of magnesium deficiency is stress. Your job, your romantic situation, your diet, your exposure to different chemicals or heavy metals—all these can act as stressors, depleting your body's natural supplies of magnesium. Identify the stressors in your life, and attempt to resolve or reduce them.

Next, learn to monitor your body's magnesium levels. You can do this by ordering a magnesium red blood cell (RBC-Mg) test. The test results will let you know if you, like most Americans, are magnesium deficient. Then, following the guidelines offered in Chapter 6, assess your magnesium burn rate (MBR), and use it to determine the amount of magnesium your body needs to function optimally. Whether by eating more magnesium-rich foods or by taking oral or topical magnesium supplements, you can quickly and easily reverse any level of magnesium deficiency you might have.

Finally, continue to monitor your magnesium levels, adjusting your intake according to the amount and intensity of stress you encounter. Because your stress levels are constantly fluctuating, your magnesium needs will also vary; depending on the kind of day you're having, you may want to take more or less magnesium. As you increase your magnesium intake, it won't be long before you notice improvements in your energy levels and your overall health, particularly where your heart is concerned. The more diligently you commit yourself to following the guidelines set forth in this book, the better the results will be.

Will a single pill cure all your health problems? Absolutely not. You must take responsibility to eat appropriately and exercise regularly. But by working with a health professional and assuming responsibility for your own well-being, you can add many happy, active years to your life.

I dream of a time when heart disease is largely a thing of the past. It is precisely this vision that has guided me as I wrote this book. I firmly believe that this dream can one day become a reality. By raising a groundswell of public awareness as to the importance of magnesium for heart health—by making it common knowledge, one person at a time—I hope to end our nation's greatest epidemic for good.

Perhaps one day, popping a magnesium supplement in the morning will be as common as taking a baby aspirin to protect yourself from a heart attack. Change begins with you, the reader. Armed with the knowledge you have gained from this book, you have all the tools you need to take the next step and build long, healthy lives for yourself and your loved ones.

If you need advice or encouragement, feel free to contact me through my website, www.dennisgoodmanmd.com. I can help— but only you can make the decision to improve your well-being with magnesium. The choice is yours.

Resources

The Author's Website: Dennis Goodman, MD, FACP, FACC, FCCP
www.dennisgoodmanmd.com
Shares important information on integrative medicine and heart health.

Additional Information on Magnesium

Jigsaw Health
15863 North Greenway-Hayden
  Loop, Suite 120
Scottsdale, AZ 85260
(480) 951–0840
(866) 601–5800
www.JigsawHealth.com
Provides extensive information on the benefits of taking magnesium; also contains resource guide to understanding many common ailments. Manufactures high-quality magnesium supplements with proprietary sustained release technology (SRT).

Magnesium Advocacy Group
www.gotmag.org
Run by former hospital executive Morley Robbins and supported by a scientific advisory board of ten acclaimed health professionals, the Magnesium Advocacy Group seeks to raise awareness and educate the public on magnesium deficiency.

The Magnesium Online Library
www.mgwater.com
Contains a comprehensive collection of articles and studies about magnesium, as well as a complete book by pioneering magnesium researcher Mildred S. Seelig, MD. Also has links to over 300 other articles about magnesium and magnesium deficiency.

The Nutritional Magnesium Association
www.nutritionalmagnesium.org
Provides up-to-date information on using nutritional magnesium for overall wellness as treatment for a number of serious health conditions, including autism, asthma, cancer, diabetes, and heart disease.

Organizations That Promote Integrative Medicine

While the physicians who belong to the following organizations place an emphasis on nutritional medicine, individual members may not be aware of the wide range of health benefits that magnesium offers. Therefore, when choosing a physician to work with, be sure to inquire about their expertise in this area.

American College for Advancement in Medicine (ACAM)
2350 Highway 138 NW
Monroe, GA 30655
(949) 309–3520
www.acamnet.org

The American College for Advancement in Medicine (ACAM) provides continuing education for doctors in complementary, integrative and alternative medicine. Their website provides many resources for patients, including a directory of ACAM members.

American Holistic Medical Association
27629 Chagrin Boulevard, Suite 206
Woodmere, OH 44122
(216) 292–6644
info@holisticmedicine.org
www.holisticmedicine.org

The American Holistic Medical Association is the oldest national organization devoted to the promotion of holistic and integrative medicine. Their website provides information on the principles and practice of holistic medicine, and includes a directory of providers who specialize in it.

Functional Medicine University (FMU)
2123 Old Spartanburg Road #348

Greer, SC 29650
(877) 328–4035
www.functionalmedicine
 university.com
www.functionalmedicine
 doctors.com

The Functional Medicine University (FMU) offers training for doctors in functional medicine, an approach to health care that uses a variety of diagnostic tests and treatments to optimize patient wellness. The first website provides resources for understanding functional medicine; the second is an online directory that will help you locate doctors who have completed the FMU training program.

The Society for Orthomolecular Health Medicine
2698 Pacific Avenue
San Francisco, CA 94115
Tel: (415) 922-6462
sohma@aol.com
www.orthomed.org

Founded by two-time Nobel Prize laureate Linus Pauling, the Society for Ortho-molecular Health Medicine promotes the practice of orthomolecular medicine, an approach to optimizing health that emphasizes restoring biochemical balance through high doses of vitamins, minerals, and hormones. A physicians' directory is available upon request.

References

Chapter 1

Go, Alan S, et al. "AHA statistical update: heart disease and stroke statistics—2013 update." *Circulation* 2013; 127(1): e6–e245.

"Heart disease facts." *CDC.gov.* Last modified March 19, 2013. www.cdc.gov/heartdisease/facts.htm.

"Periodontal disease and atherosclerotic vascular disease: does the evidence support an independent association?" *Heart.org.* Last modified May 15, 2012. http://newsroom.heart.org/news/periodontal-disease-and-atherosclerotic-234243.

Chapter 2

Cohen, Suzy. *Drug Muggers: Which Medications Are Robbing Your Body of Essential Nutrients-And Natural Ways To Restore Them.* Emmaus, PA: Rodale Books, 2011.

David, DR, et al. "Changes in USDA food composition data for 43 garden crops, 1950–1999." *J Amer Coll Nutr* 2004; 23(6):669–682.

Flink, EB. "Magnesium deficiency–etiology and clinical spectrum." *Acta Med. Scand. Suppl.* 1981; 209(S647):125–37.

Huber, DM. "The Woes of GMOs - Glyphosate and GMOs' impact on crops, soils, animals and man." *GM Watch.* Last modified Sept. 3, 2012. www.gmwatch.org/latest-listing/51–2012/14164-glyphosate-and-gmos-impact-on-crops-soils-animals-and-man-dr-don-huber.

Larsson, S, et al. "Dietary magnesium intake and risk of stroke: a meta-analysis of prospective studies." *Am J Clin Nutr.* 2012; 95(2): 269–270.

Marler, JB, et al. "Human health, the nutritional quality of harvested food and sustainable farming systems." *Nutritionsecurity.org* Last modified 2006. www.nutritionsecurity.org/PDF/NSI_White%20Paper_Web.pdf.

Piovesan, D, et al. "The human 'magnesome': detecting magnesium binding sites on human proteins." *BMC Bioinformatics* 2012; 13 (Suppl 14):S10.

Pitkänen, H. "Industrial possibilities to interfere with the salt problem: dietary Na/(K+Mg) ratio." *Magnesium* 1982;1:298–303.

Spiroux de Vendômois, J, et al. "A comparison of the effects of three GM corn varieties on mammalian health." *Int J Biol Sci* 2009; 5(7):706–726.

Chapter 3

"About heart failure." *Heart.org*. Last modified August 20, 2012. www.heart .org/HEARTORG/Conditions/HeartFailure/AboutHeartFailure/About-Heart-Failure_UCM_002044_Article.jsp.

"Anatomy of the heart." *Texasheartinstitute.org*. Last modified August 2012. www.texasheartinstitute.org/HIC/Anatomy/anatomy2.cfm.

Iseri, LT, et al. "Magnesium: nature's physiologic calcium blocker." *Am Heart J* 1984; 108(1): 188–193.

"What is an arrhythmia?" *NHBLI.NIH.gov*. Last modified July 1, 2011. www.nhlbi.nih.gov/health/health-topics/topics/arr/

"What is the heart? *NHBLI.NIH.gov*. Last modified November 17, 2011. www.nhlbi.nih.gov/health/health-topics/topics/hhw/.

"Your heart and blood vessels." *My.ClevelandClinic.org*. Last modified 2013. http://my.clevelandclinic.org/heart/heartworks/heartfacts.aspx.

Chapter 4

Altura, BM, et al. "Cardiovascular risk factors and magnesium: relationships to artherosclerosis, ischemic heart disease and hypertension." *Magnes Trace Elem* 1991–92; 10(2–4):182–192.

—. "Short term Mg deficiency results in decreased levels of serum sphingomyelin, lipid peroxidation, and apoptosis in cardiovascular tissues." *Am J Phys Heart Circ Physiol* 2009; 297(1): H86–92.

Baigent, C, et al. "Efficacy and safety of cholesterol-lowering treatment: prospective meta-analysis of data from 90,056 participants in 14 randomised trials of statins. *Lancet.* 2005;366:1267–1278.

Cohen, Jay S. *The Magnesium Solution for High Blood Pressure.* Garden City Park, NY: Square One Publishers, 2004.

Del Gobbo, L, et al. "Circulating and dietary magnesium and risk of cardio-vascular disease: a systematic review and meta-analysis of prospective studies." *Amer J Clin Nutr* 2013; 98(1):160–173.

Durlach, J. "Clinical aspects of chronic magnesium deficiency." In *Magnesium in Health and Disease,* edited by Mildred Seelig, 883–909. New York, Spectrum Publications, 1980.

Durlach, J, et al. "Magnesium and therapeutics." *Magnes Res* 1994; 7(3/4): 313–28.

Falk, E, et al. "Coronary Plaque Disruption." *Circulation* 1995; 92(3): 657–671.

Fuster, V, ed. *The Vulnerable Artherosclerotic Plaque: Understanding, Identification and Modification.* Austin, TX: Futura Publishing, 1998.

Haga, H. "Effects of dietary magnesium supplementation on diurnal variations of blood pressure and plasma sodium, potassium-ATPase activity in essential hypertension." *Japan Heart Journal* 1992;33(6):785–800.

Joosten, MM et al. "Urinary magnesium excretion and risk of hypertension: the prevention of renal and vascular end-stage disease study." *Hypertension* 2013;61(6):1161–7.

—. "Urinary and plasma magnesium and risk of ischemic heart disease." *Amer J of Clin Nutr* 2013; 97(6):1299–306.

Karppanen, H, et al. "Minerals, coronary heart disease and sudden coronary death." *Advances in Cardiology* 1978; 25:9–24.

Liao, F, et al. "Is low magnesium concentration a risk factor for coronary heart disease? The Atherosclerosis Risk in Communities (ARIC) Study." *American heart journal* 1998; 136(3):480–490.

Libby, P. "Atherosclerosis: The New View." *Sci Am* 2002; 286(5):47–58.

Libby, P, et al. "Inflammation and atherosclerosis." *Circulation* 2002; 105(9) 1135–1143.

Maier, JAM. "Endothelial cells and magnesium: implications in atherosclerosis." *Clinical Science* 2012; 122(9):397–407.

Malpuech-Brugère, C, et al. "Exacerbated immune stress response during experimental magnesium deficiency results from abnormal cell calcium homeostasis." *Life Sciences* 1998; 63(20):1815–1822.

Mann, George V, ed. *Coronary Heart Disease: The Dietary Sense and Nonsense.* New York: Veritas Society, 1993.

Naghavi, M, et al. "From vulnerable plaque to vulnerable patient: a call for new definitions and risk assessment strategies: part 1." *Circulation* 2003; 108(14): 1664–1672.

Peacock, JM, et al. "Serum magnesium and risk of sudden cardiac death in the Atherosclerosis Risk in Communities (ARIC) Study." *Amer Heart J* 2010;160(3):464–470.

Ray, KK, et al. "Statins and all-cause mortality in high-risk primary prevention: a meta-analysis of 11 randomized controlled trials involving 65,299 participants." *Arch Intern Med* 2010;170(12):1024–31.

Resnick, LM. "Magnesium in the pathophysiology and treatment of hypertension & diabetes mellitus: where are we in 1997? *Am J of Hypertension* 1997;10(3):368–370.

Rosanoff, A. "Rising Ca:Mg intake ratio from food in USA Adults: a concern." *Magnes Res* 2010; 23(4): 181–193.

Rude, RK, et al. "Skeletal and hormonal effects of magnesium deficiency." *J Amer Coll of Nutr* 2009; 28(2):131–141.

Seelig, Mildred S. *Magnesium Deficiency in the Pathogenesis of Disease.* New York: Plenum Publishing, 1980.

Seelig, Mildred, and Andrea Rosanoff. *The Magnesium Factor.* New York: Avery, 2003.

Selye, H. *Calciphylaxis.* Chicago, IL: The University of Chicago Press, 1962.

—. "The chemical prevention of cardiac necrosis." *Amer J of Medical Sciences.* Jul 1959; 238(1):130.

Stary, H, et al. "A definition of advanced types of atherosclerotic lesions and a histological classification of atherosclerosis." *Arteriosclerosis, Thrombosis, and Vascular Biology* 1995; 15(9):1512–1531.

Thavendiranathan, P, et al. "Primary prevention of cardiovascular disease with statin therapy." *Arch Intern Med* 2006;166(21):2307–13.

Weglicki, WB. "Hypomagnesemia and inflammation: clinical and basic aspects." *Annu Rev Nutr* 2012;32:55–71.

Weglicki, et al. "Pathobiology of magnesium deficiency: a cytokine/neurogenic inflammation hypothesis." *AJP—Regu Physiol* 1992; 263(3):R734–R737.

Weglicki, WB, et al. "The role of magnesium deficiency in cardiovascular and intestinal inflammation." *Magnes Res* 2010; 23(4):S199–S206.

Wolf, FI, et al. "Magnesium deficiency and endothelial dysfunction: is oxidative stress involved?" *Magnes Res* 2008; 21(1): 58–64.

Chapter 5

Abraham, GE, et al. "Serum and red cell magnesium levels in patients with premenstrual tension." *Am J Clin Nutr.* 1981; 34(11):2364–2366.

Bagis, S, et al. "Is magnesium citrate treatment effective on pain, clinical parameters, and functional status in patients with fibromyalgia?" *Rheumatol Int.* 2013; 33(1):167–172.

Bendich, A. "The potential for dietary supplements to reduce premenstrual syndrome (PMS) symptoms." *J Am Coll Nutr* 2000; 19(1):3–12.

Blitz, M, et al. "Aerosolized magnesium sulfate for acute asthma." *Chest* 2005; 128(1):337–344.

Cox, IM, et al. "Red blood cell magnesium and chronic fatigue syndrome." *Lancet* 1991;337(8744):757–60.

Deans, Emily. "Magnesium and the brain: the original chill pill." *Psychology-Today.com.* http://www.psychologytoday.com/blog/evolutionary-psychiatry/201106/magnesium-and-the-brain-the-original-chill-pill.

Eby, GA, et al. "Hypothesis for magnesium depletion, calcium and glutamate overload as cause of most major depression and related mental health issues: a review of the neurobiochemistry, animal and human evidence with a suggested treatment protocol." *George-eby-research.com.* Last modified December 2008. george-eby-research.com/html/depression-treatment-dec-2008.doc.

—. "Magnesium for treatment-resistant depression: a review and hypothesis." *Med Hypotheses* 2010; 74(4):649–660.

—. "Rapid recovery from major depression using magnesium treatment." *Med Hypotheses* 2006;67(2):362–370.

Elisaf, M, et al. "Hypomagnesemic hypokalemia and hypocalcemia: clinical and laboratory characteristics." *Mineral Electrolyte Metab* 1997;23(2):105–112.

Facchinetti, F, et al. "Oral magnesium successfully relieves premenstrual mood changes." *Obstet Gynocol* 1991;78(2):177–181.

Guerrero-Romero, F and M Rodriguez-Moran. "Low serum magnesium levels in metabolic syndrome." *Acta Diabetologica* 2002; 39(4):209–213.

Guerrera, MP, et al. "Therapeutic uses of magnesium." *Am Fam Physician* 2009;80(2):157–62.

Gilliland, FD, et al. "Dietary magnesium, potassium, sodium, and children's lung function." *Amer J Epidemiol* 2002;155(2):125–131.

Gontijo-Amaral, C, et al. "Oral magnesium supplementation in asthmatic children: a double-blind randomized placebo-controlled trial." *Eur J Clin Nutr* 2007;61(1):54–60.

Hashimoto, Y, et al. "Assessment of magnesium status in patients with bronchial asthma." *J Asthma* 2000;37(6):489–496.

He, K, et al. "Magnesium intake and incidence of metabolic syndrome among young adults." *Circulation* 2006;113(13):1675–1682.

Huerta, MG, et al. "Magnesium deficiency is associated with insulin resistance in obese children." *Diabetes Care*. 2005; 28(5):1175–1181.

Johanson, JF. "Review of the treatment options for chronic constipation." *MedGenMed*. 2007; 9(2):25.

Johansson, G, et al. "Effects of magnesium hydroxide in renal stone disease." *J Am Coll Nutr*. 1982;1(2):179–185.

Kazaks, AG, et al. "Effect of oral magnesium supplementation on measures of airway resistance and subjective assessment of asthma control and quality of life in men and women with mild to moderate asthma: a randomized placebo controlled trial." *J Asthma* 2010; 47(1):83–92.

Ladefoged, K, et al. "Nutrition in short-bowel syndrome." *Scand J Gastroenterol Suppl* 1996;216:122–131.

Lopez-Ridaura, R, et al. "Magnesium intake and risk of type 2 diabetes in men and women." *Diabetes Care* 2004; 27(1):134–140.

Mauskop, Alexander and Barry Fox. *What Your Doctor May Not Tell You About Migraines*. New York: Warner Books, 2001.

Mozumdar, A, and G Liquori. "Persistent increase of prevalence of metabolic syndrome among us adults: NHANES III to NHANES 1999–2006." *Diabetes Care*. 2011; 34(1):216–219.

Nadler, JL, et al. "Magnesium deficiency produces insulin resistance and increased thromboxane synthesis." *Hypertension* 1993;21(6 pt 2):1024–1029.

Nielsen FH. "Magnesium, inflammation, and obesity in chronic disease." *Nutr Rev* 2010; 68(6):333–340.

Nielsen, FH, et al. "Magnesium supplementation improves indicators of low magnesium status and inflammatory stress in adults older than 51 years with poor quality sleep." *Magnes Res* 2010; 23(4):158–168.

Paolisso, G, et al. "Magnesium and glucose homeostasis." *Diabetologia* 1990; 33(9):511–514.

Park, JH, et al. "Use of P-31 magnetic resonance spectroscopy to detect metabolic abnormalities in muscles of patients with fibromyalgia." *Arthritis Rheum* 1998; 41(3):406–413.

Prien, EL, and SN Gershoff. "Magnesium oxide-pyridoxine therapy for recurrent calcium oxalate calculi." *J Urol* 1974; 112(4):509–512.

Rayssiguier, Y et al. "Magnesium deficiency and metabolic syndrome: stress and inflammation may reflect calcium activation." *Magnes Res* 2010;23 (2):73–80.

Rodríguez-Morán, M, and F Guerrero-Romero. "Oral magnesium supplementation improves insulin sensitivity and metabolic control in type 2 diabetic subjects: a randomized double-blind controlled trial." *Diabetes Care* 2003; 26(4):1147–1152.

Rude, Robert K. and Maurice E. Shils. "Magnesium." In *Modern Nutrition in Health and Disease,* edited by Shils, Moshe Shike, A. Catharine Ross, Benjamin Caballero, Robert J. Cousins, 223–247. Baltimore, MD: Lippincott Williams & Wilkins, 2006.

Ryder, KM, et al. "Magnesium intake from food and supplements is associated with bone mineral density in healthy older white subjects." *J Am Geriatr Soc* 200; 53(11):1875–1880.

Tucker, KL, et al. "Potassium, magnesium, and fruit and vegetable intakes are associated with greater bone mineral density in elderly men and women." *Am J Clin Nutr* 1999; 69(4):727–736.

Walker, AF, et al. "Magnesium supplementation alleviates premenstrual symptoms of fluid retention." *J Womens Health* 1998;7(9):1157–1165.

White, JR, and RK Campbell. "Magnesium and diabetes: a review." *Ann Pharmacother* 1993; 27(6):775–780.

Wright, Jonathan V. and Alan R. Gaby. *Natural Medicine, Optimal Wellness.* Garden City Park, NY: Square One Publishers, 2006.

Chapter 6

Krebs-Smith. SM. "Americans do not meet federal dietary recommendations." *J of Nutr.* 2010; 140(10):1832–1838.

"Magnesium: Health Professional Fact Sheet." *NIH.gov.* Last modified July 13, 2009. http://ods.od.nih.gov/factsheets/Magnesium-HealthProfessional/.

Seelig, MS. "The requirement of magnesium by the normal adult." *Amer J of Clin Nutr* 1964; 14(6): 342–390.

About the Author

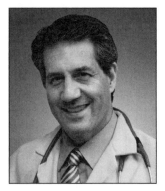

Dr. Dennis Goodman, MD, FACC, graduated cum laude and with distinction from the University of Cape Town Medical School in Cape Town, South Africa, in 1979. He served his internship at Grootte Schuur Hospital in Cape Town, South Africa, and completed his internal medicine residency at Montefiore Hospital in Pittsburgh, Pennsylvania, where he was also Chief Medical Resident. Dr. Goodman served his cardiology fellowship at Baylor College of Medicine in Houston, Texas.

Dr. Goodman is board certified in internal medicine, cardiology, interventional cardiology, clinical lipidology, critical care, integrative holistic and integrative medicine, and cardiac CT imaging. In 1988, he joined Scripps Memorial Hospital in La Jolla, California, where he served as Chief of Cardiology and Medical Director of Cardiac Rehabilitation. In 2009 he joined the New York University cardiology faculty and was appointed Director of Chest Pain at Bellevue Hospital in New York.

Currently, Dr. Goodman is a Clinical Associate Professor of Medicine at New York University. He is also a faculty member of Leon H. Charney Division of Cardiology and Preventative Medicine at NYU, as well as the Director of Integrative Medicine. His area of special interest lies in the prevention, early detection, and treatment of cardiovascular disease with an integrative approach to optimal patient health care.

The author of three books on heart health, Dr. Goodman is a noted international speaker and has been a visiting teaching professor throughout Europe, Asia, South Africa, Israel, and the United Kingdom. His articles have been widely published, and he has appeared on numerous radio and television programs on such major networks as FOX, ABC, CBS, and NBC. Dr. Goodman has been consistently listed among New York's Top Physicians and Cardiologists.

Index

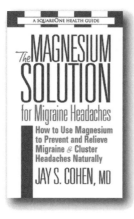

THE MAGNESIUM SOLUTION FOR MIGRAINE HEADACHES

How to Use Magnesium to Prevent and Relieve Migraine & Cluster Headaches Naturally

Jay S. Cohen, MD

More than 30 million people across North America suffer from migraine headaches. While a number of drugs are used to treat migraines, these treatments don't work for everyone and come with a high risk of side effects. Fortunately, Dr. Jay S. Cohen has discovered an alternative—magnesium.

This easy-to-understand guide explains what migraines are, and shows how magnesium can play a role in preventing and treating them. It also pinpoints the best magnesium to use, as well as the proper dosage to prevent or stop migraines. For those looking for a safe and effective approach to migraine and cluster headaches, Dr. Cohen prescribes a proven remedy in *The Magnesium Solution for Migraine Headaches.*

$5.95 US • 96 pages • 4 x 7-inch mass paperback • ISBN 978-0-7570-0256-4

THE MAGNESIUM SOLUTION FOR HIGH BLOOD PRESSURE

How to Use Magnesium to Help Prevent & Relieve Hypertension Naturally

Jay S. Cohen, MD

Approximately 50 percent of Americans have hypertension, a condition that can lead to hardening of the arteries, heart attack, and stroke. While many medications are available to combat this condition, these drugs come with potentially dangerous side effects. When Dr. Jay S. Cohen learned of his own hypertension, he was aware of the risks associated with standard treatments and selected a safer option—magnesium.

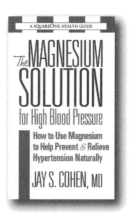

In *The Magnesium Solution for High Blood Pressure,* Dr. Cohen describes the best types of magnesium for treating hypertension, explores appropriate dosage, and details the use of magnesium with hypertension meds. Here is a proven remedy for anyone looking for a safe, effective approach to high blood pressure.

$5.95 US • 96 pages • 4 x 7-inch mass paperback • ISBN 978-0-7570-0255-7

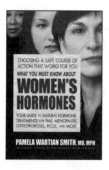

WHAT YOU MUST KNOW ABOUT
WOMEN'S HORMONES
Your Guide to Natural Hormone Treatments for PMS, Menopause, Osteoporosis, PCOS, and More
Pamela Wartian Smith, MD, MPH

Hormonal imbalances can occur at any age and for a variety of reasons. While most related problems are associated with menopause, fluctuating hormonal levels can also cause a variety of other conditions. *What You Must Know About Women's Hormones* is a guide to the treatment of hormonal irregularities without the health risks associated with standard hormone replacement therapy.

Part I of this book describes the body's own hormones, looking at their functions and the problems that can occur if they are not at optimal levels. Part II focuses on the most common problems that arise from hormonal imbalances, such as PMS and endometriosis. Part III details hormone replacement therapy, focusing on the difference between natural and synthetic treatments. *What You Must Know About Women's Hormones* can make a profound difference in your life.

$17.95 US • 256 pages • 6 x 9-inch quality paperback • ISBN 978-0-7570-0307-3

WHAT YOU MUST KNOW ABOUT
BIOIDENTICAL HORMONE REPLACEMENT THERAPY
An Alternative Approach to Effectively Treating the Symptoms of Menopause
Amy Lee Hawkins, PharmD

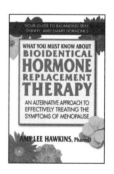

Although normal and natural, menopause can cause severe symptoms, ranging from insomnia and hot flashes to anxiety and depression. Because standard hormone replacement therapy can increase the risk of heart attack, stroke, breast cancer, and blood clots, women often choose to go untreated even when menopausal problems have a profound impact on their lives--or they did, until now. In her new book, Dr. Amy Lee Hawkins offers real help through a lesser-known approach called *bioidentical hormone replacement therapy* (BHRT)—a treatment that can help diminish menopausal symptoms without the dangers of synthetic drugs.

If you are struggling with menopause-related problems, you want the safest, most effective route to feeling better. *What You Must Know About Bioidentical Hormone Replacement Therapy* provides the information you need to make the best possible decisions about your health.

$17.95 US • 240 pages • 6 x 9-inch quality paperback • ISBN 978-0-7570-0380-6